About the NCCN Guidelines for Patients®

National Comprehensive Cancer Network®

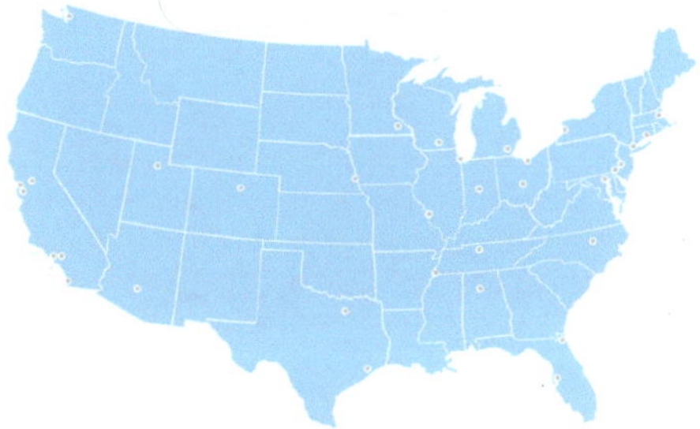

Did you know that top cancer centers across the United States work together to improve cancer care? This alliance of leading cancer centers is called the National Comprehensive Cancer Network® (NCCN®).

Cancer care is always changing. NCCN develops evidence-based cancer care recommendations used by health care providers worldwide. These frequently updated recommendations are the NCCN Clinical Practice Guidelines in Oncology (NCCN Guidelines®). The NCCN Guidelines for Patients plainly explain these expert recommendations for people with cancer and caregivers.

These NCCN Guidelines for Patients are based on the NCCN Clinical Practice Guidelines in Oncology (NCCN Guidelines®) for Esophageal and Esophagogastric Junction Cancers, Version 2.2024 – April 23, 2024

View the NCCN Guidelines for Patients free online
NCCN.org/patientguidelines

Find an NCCN Cancer Center near you
NCCN.org/cancercenters

Connect with us

Supporters

NATIONAL COMPREHENSIVE CANCER NETWORK®
NCCN FOUNDATION
Guiding Treatment. Changing Lives.

NCCN Guidelines for Patients are supported by funding from the NCCN Foundation®

NCCN Foundation gratefully acknowledges the following corporate supporters for helping to make available these NCCN Guidelines for Patients: AstraZeneca and Bristol Myers Squibb.

NCCN independently adapts, updates, and hosts the NCCN Guidelines for Patients. Our corporate supporters do not participate in the development of the NCCN Guidelines for Patients and are not responsible for the content and recommendations contained therein.

Additional support is provided by

EC Aware

ECEF ESOPHAGEAL CANCER EDUCATION FOUNDATION

Esophageal Cancer Awareness Association (ECAA) dba EC Aware

ECAA is a 501(c)(3) all-volunteer non-profit organization with four mission goals: to raise public and professional awareness of esophageal cancer; to educate the public regarding the risks and symptoms of EC; to contribute to research into detection, treatment, and cure; and to provide personal support to patients, caregivers, and loved ones. 1.800.601.0613

Esophageal Cancer Education Foundation

ECEF's mission is to bring awareness and educate the public and medical community about Esophageal Cancer and to walk the journey with patients who have this disease and to support research projects dealing with Esophageal Cancer. ECEF has developed an array of services that can assist the patient and caregiver through the esophageal cancer journey. 732.385.7461

To make a gift or learn more, visit online or email

NCCNFoundation.org/donate

PatientGuidelines@NCCN.org

Contents

NCCN Foundation seeks to support the millions of patients and their families affected by a cancer diagnosis by funding and distributing NCCN Guidelines for Patients. NCCN Foundation is also committed to advancing cancer treatment by funding the nation's promising doctors at the center of innovation in cancer research. For more details and the full library of patient and caregiver resources, visit NCCN.org/patients.

National Comprehensive Cancer Network (NCCN) and NCCN Foundation
3025 Chemical Road, Suite 100, Plymouth Meeting, PA 19462 USA

1

Esophageal cancer basics

The esophagus is a long, muscular tube through which food passes from the throat to the stomach. Esophageal cancer starts when abnormal cells grow out of control in the layers of the esophagus inner lining.

The esophagus

The esophagus is located behind the trachea (windpipe) and in front of the spine. It is part of the digestive system. The digestive system transports and breaks down food, absorbs nutrients, and removes waste from the body. It includes the esophagus, stomach, liver, pancreas, small intestine, colon, rectum, and anus.

Food and drink enter the mouth and move through the esophagus into the stomach. When you swallow, small contractions, called peristalsis, along with gravity and pressure, move food down the esophagus and into the stomach. Except during the act of swallowing, the esophagus is normally empty.

The esophagus is about 10 inches long and about 1 inch wide. It has two sphincters, circular muscles that normally remain closed except during the act of swallowing. One sphincter is located at the top of the esophagus and the other at the bottom, between the esophagus and the stomach.

The digestive tract

The digestive or gastrointestinal (GI) tract is part of the digestive system. Food enters the mouth and passes through the esophagus into the stomach. After being broken down into a liquid, food enters the small intestine. The large intestine prepares unused food to be moved out of the body.

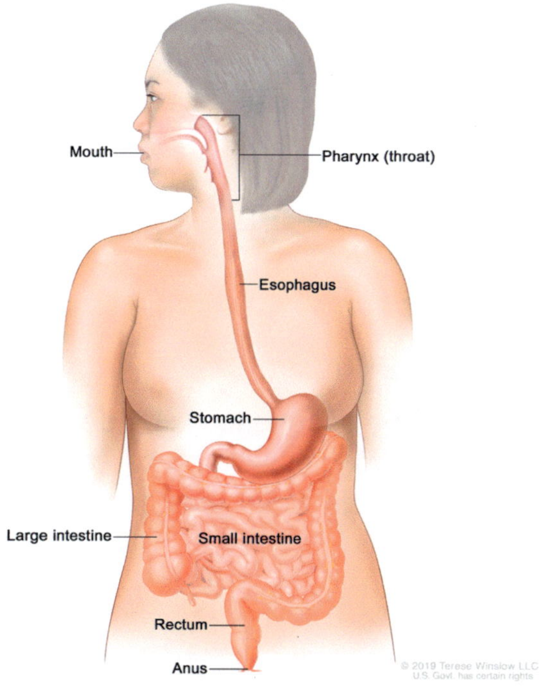

Parts of the esophagus

Esophagus wall

The esophagus wall contains 4 layers:

1. Mucosa – inner membrane that is in contact with food. It has 3 parts:
    - Epithelium – innermost lining and is normally made up of flat, thin cells called squamous cells
    - Lamina propria – thin layer of connective tissue under the epithelium
    - Muscularis mucosa - very thin layer of muscle under the lamina propria
2. Submucosa – layer of connective tissue just below the mucosa that contains blood vessels, nerves, and lymphatic vessels. In some parts of the esophagus, this layer also includes glands that secrete mucus.
3. Muscularis propria – thick layer of muscle under the submucosa. It contracts in a coordinated way to push food down the esophagus from the throat to the stomach (peristalsis).
4. Tunica adventitia – outermost layer, made of connective tissue

Upper esophagus

The upper part of the esophagus is made of striated muscle. Striated muscle generates force and contracts. It is under your control (voluntary).

Middle esophagus

The middle part of the esophagus is a mixture of striated and smooth muscle.

Lower esophagus

The lower part of the esophagus consists only of smooth muscle. Smooth muscle is not under your control. It is involuntary, like a reflex.

Esophagogastric junction

The esophagogastric junction (EGJ) is the place where the stomach and the esophagus meet, found just beneath the diaphragm. It is also called the gastroesophageal junction (GEJ). It separates the contents of the esophagus from the contents of the stomach (acid).

Esophageal cancer

Cancer of the esophagus (or esophageal cancer) starts when cells in the epithelium of the esophagus begin to grow out of control.

There are 2 types of esophageal cancer:

- **Esophageal squamous cell carcinoma (ESCC)** starts in the thin, flat cells found in the inner lining of the esophagus. Squamous cell carcinoma (SCC) is often found in the upper and middle esophagus but can occur in the lower esophagus as well.
- **Esophageal adenocarcinoma (EAC)** starts in the mucus-making cells of the inner lining of the esophagus. Adenocarcinomas are often found in the

lower esophagus but can occur in the middle esophagus as well.

Today, most esophageal cancers in North America and Western Europe are adenocarcinomas. Squamous cell carcinoma is more common in Eastern Europe, Asia, and Africa. Treatment is based on the type and location of esophageal cancer, in addition to the stage of the tumor (where it is in the body).

Some tumors that start in the stomach and cross over into the area between the esophagus and stomach (esophagogastric junction) are treated as esophageal cancers and not as stomach cancers. However, this depends on the exact location of the tumor. Siewert types used as part of cancer staging describe where the tumor is relative to the esophagus and stomach.

Barrett esophagus

In Barrett esophagus (BE), the squamous cells that line the lower part of the esophagus have changed or been replaced with abnormal cells as a result of chronic reflux. Those with Barrett esophagus are at risk of developing adenocarcinoma of the esophagus.

How cancer spreads

Esophageal cancer usually starts in the innermost layer (mucosa) and grows outward through and along the layers of the esophagus wall. Cancer can spread to nearby lymph nodes, veins, arteries, and organs such as the liver, pancreas, lung, and spleen. It might also grow into nearby lymphatic or blood vessels, and from there spread to nearby lymph nodes or to other parts of the body.

Through your cancer care, you might find measurements using the metric system (centimeters, millimeters, etc.). That is because your care team uses the metric system to measure many aspects of treatment.

Esophageal cancers tend to develop slowly over many years. Before cancer develops, precancerous changes often occur in the inner lining (mucosa) of the esophagus. Since these early changes rarely cause symptoms, they often go undetected.

Stages of esophageal cancer can be grouped into 3 main categories, depending on how far the cancer has spread.

- **Early-stage cancer** has not grown beyond the inside of the esophagus. The tumor may be very small (2 centimeters or less, which is about the size of a peanut) and is not in any lymph nodes.
- **Locoregional or locally advanced** cancer has invaded the esophagus wall and/or spread to the lymph nodes or organs near or in direct contact with the esophagus.
- **Metastatic cancer** has spread to other parts of the body. The most common metastatic sites are the liver, distant lymph nodes, lung, bone, and brain.

Key points

- Most esophageal cancers start in cells that line the inside of the esophagus and secrete mucus. These esophageal cancers are called adenocarcinomas.
- Esophageal squamous cell carcinoma starts in the thin, flat cells found in the inner lining of the esophagus.
- The esophagus wall is made up of 4 main layers: mucosa, submucosa, muscularis propria, and tunica adventitia.
- Esophageal cancers tend to develop slowly over many years. Before cancer develops, pre-cancerous changes often occur in the inner lining (mucosa) of the esophagus.
- Early-stage esophageal cancer is contained in the esophagus. The tumor is often small and is not in any lymph nodes.
- Locoregional or locally advanced esophageal cancer has invaded other layers of the esophagus wall and/or spread to the lymph nodes or organs near or in direct contact with the esophagus.
- Cancer can spread to distant parts of the body through the blood or lymphatic system. This is called metastatic esophageal cancer. Distant metastases could be in the liver, distant lymph nodes, and lung.

2
Diagnosing esophageal cancer

Treatment planning starts with testing. This chapter presents an overview of the tests you might receive and what to expect.

Test results

Results from blood tests, imaging studies, and biopsy will be used to determine your treatment plan. It is important you understand what these tests mean. Ask questions and keep copies of your test results. Online patient portals are one way to access your test results.

Keep these things in mind:

- It's beneficial to have a support system in place during diagnosis and treatment. Enlist the help of friends, family members, or peers who can provide transportation, meals, and emotional support. These can be different people for different tasks or change over time.
- Bring someone with you to doctor visits, if possible.
- Write down questions and take notes during appointments. Don't be afraid to ask your care team questions. Get to know your care team and help them get to know you.
- Get copies of blood tests, imaging results, and reports about the specific type of cancer you have.
- Organize your papers. Create files for insurance forms, medical records, and test results. You can do the same on your computer.
- Keep a list of contact information for everyone on your care team. Add it to your phone. Hang the list on your refrigerator or keep it in a place where someone can access it in an emergency. Keep your primary care physician informed of changes to this list.
- In your contact list, include information on your exact type of cancer, as well as any treatments and the date each treatment started.
- Set up an online patient portal (MyChart or health record account) if it's available, which can help you track your appointments and communicate with your care team. Remember, many times, the portal messages are not immediately seen by a nurse or physician. Be sure to ask your care team how best to communicate with them, especially in an emergency.

More information on these tests is on the following pages. For possible tests, **see Guide 1.**

Guide 1 **Possible tests for esophageal cancer**
Medical history and physical exam. Screen for family history
Upper GI endoscopy and biopsy
CT of chest/abdomen with oral and IV contrast. CT of pelvis with contrast as needed
FDG-PET/CT evaluation (skull base to mid-thigh) if no evidence of metastatic disease
Complete blood count (CBC) and comprehensive chemistry profile
Endoscopic ultrasound (EUS) if no evidence of metastatic unresectable disease
Endoscopic resection (ER) is recommended for the accurate staging of early-stage cancers (T1a or T1b). Early-stage cancers can best be diagnosed by ER.
Biopsy of metastatic disease as needed
Tumor testing for microsatellite instability (MSI) or mismatch repair (MMR) is recommended in all newly diagnosed patients
PD-L1 testing if advanced/metastatic disease is suspected
HER2 testing if metastatic adenocarcinoma is suspected
Bronchoscopy, if tumor is at or above the carina (the ridge at the base of the trachea) with no evidence of metastatic disease
Assign Siewert category
Nutritional assessment and counseling
Smoking cessation advice, counseling, and medicine as needed

General health tests

Medical history

A medical history is a record of all health issues and treatments you have had in your life. Be prepared to list any illness or injury and when it happened. Bring a list of old and new medicines and any over-the-counter medicines, herbals, or supplements you take. Tell your doctor about any symptoms you have. A medical (or health) history will help determine which treatment is best for you.

Family history

Some cancers and other diseases can run in families. Your doctor will ask about the health history of family members who are blood relatives. This information is called a family history. You can ask family members about their health issues like heart disease, cancer, and diabetes, and at what age they were diagnosed.

Physical exam

During a physical exam, your doctor may:

- Check your temperature, blood pressure, pulse, and breathing rate
- Check your weight
- Listen to your lungs and heart
- Look in your eyes, ears, nose, and throat
- Feel and apply pressure to parts of your body to see if organs are of normal size, are soft or hard, or cause pain when touched
- Feel for enlarged lymph nodes in your neck, underarm, and groin

Nutritional assessment

You may need to meet with a nutrition expert before starting treatment. The nutritionist or dietician can assess the impact of the cancer on your health. Esophageal cancer can make you lose your appetite or cause difficulty or pain when swallowing foods or liquids. You may also feel full after eating very little. These changes may have caused you to lose too much weight or make you feel weak and tired.

It is important that you receive adequate and sustained nutrition before you start treatment. You might receive food through a plastic tube that is placed through the skin of your abdomen into your stomach or small intestine.

During and after treatment, your care team will monitor for weight loss and other signs you aren't getting enough nutrition.

Blood tests

Blood tests check for signs of disease and how well organs are working. They require a sample of your blood, which is removed through a needle placed into your vein.

Complete blood count

A complete blood count (CBC) measures the levels of red blood cells, white blood cells, and platelets in your blood. Your doctor will want to know if you have enough red blood cells to carry oxygen throughout your body, white blood cells to fight infection, and platelets to control bleeding.

Comprehensive chemistry profile

A comprehensive chemistry profile provides important information about how well your kidneys and liver are working, among other things. It is usually part of a comprehensive metabolic panel (CMP). A CMP measures 14 different substances in your blood.

Nutrition matters

Esophageal cancer can make eating more challenging. A dietician or nutritionist can help you with any nutrition needs before, during, and after cancer treatment.

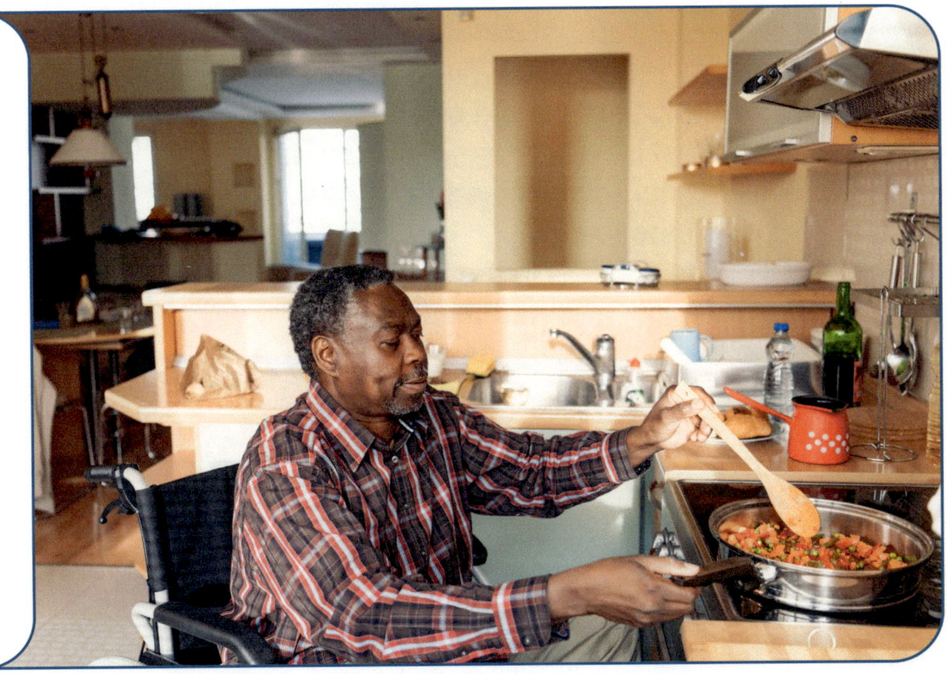

Imaging tests

Imaging tests take pictures of the inside of your body. Images can be made with scanning machines or scoping tools. Imaging tests may show if the tumor involves any veins, arteries, and other organs. A radiologist, an expert in interpreting imaging tests, will write a report and send this report to your doctor. Your doctor will discuss the results with you.

CT scan

A computed tomography (CT or CAT) scan uses x-rays and computer technology to take pictures of the inside of the body. It takes many x-rays of the same body part from different angles. All the images are combined to make one detailed three-dimensional (3D) picture.

A CT scan of your chest, abdomen, and/or pelvis may be one of the tests to look for cancer. Oral (by mouth) and IV (by a needle placed into a vein in your arm) contrast are often used together when testing for esophageal cancer.

Contrast materials are not dyes, but substances that help to make the pictures clearer. The contrast is not permanent and will leave the body in your urine immediately after the test. Tell your care team if you have had allergic reactions to contrast in the past. This is important. You might be given medicines to avoid the effects of those allergies.

PET scan

A positron emission tomography (PET) scan uses a radioactive drug called a tracer that is not harmful. A tracer is a substance injected into a vein to see where cancer cells are in the body and if they are using sugar produced by your body to grow. Cancer cells show up as bright spots on PET scans. However, not all tumors will appear on a PET scan. Also, not all bright spots are cancer. It is normal for the brain, heart, kidneys, and bladder to be bright on a PET scan. Inflammation or infection can also show up as a bright spot. When a PET scan is combined with CT, it is called a PET/CT scan. It may be done with one or two machines depending on the cancer center. An FDG-PET/CT scan uses 18-fluorodeoxyglucose as its tracer.

Ultrasound

An ultrasound (US) uses high-energy sound waves to form pictures of the inside of the body. This is similar to the sonogram used for pregnancy. A wand-like probe (transducer) will be held and pressed onto your abdomen using gel. Ultrasound does not use x-rays. It can show small areas of cancer that are near the skin. Sometimes, an ultrasound or CT is used to guide a biopsy.

Endoscopy procedures

Some imaging tests use a thin, tube-shaped tool called a scope that is inserted into the body to take pictures. One end of the scope has a small light and camera lens to see inside your body. The image is sent to a television monitor. This will help guide your doctor in a biopsy, stent placement, or other tasks. The scope is guided into the body through a natural opening, such as the mouth, nose, or anus. It may also be inserted through a small surgical cut.

More than one type of scope may be used for imaging tests. The type of scope often used for esophageal cancer is called an endoscope. An endoscope is often guided into the body through the mouth. Endoscopy is an important tool in the diagnosis, staging, treatment, and care of those with esophageal cancer. Before an endoscopy, you will be given medicine to help you relax or sleep during the procedure.

Endoscopic ultrasound

Endoscopic ultrasound (EUS) uses both imaging and an endoscope to see how deep the tumor has grown into the esophagus wall. Signs of cancer within lymph nodes and other nearby organs can also be detected. An EUS is an important part of cancer diagnosis and staging.

Upper GI endoscopy or EGD

In an upper gastrointestinal (GI) endoscopy or esophagogastroduodenoscopy (EGD), a device is guided down the throat into the esophagus, stomach, and upper parts of the small intestine (duodenum). An EGD is used to inspect the lining of these organs and to look for any signs of cancer or other abnormalities such as dilated blood vessels or ulcers. Biopsies are usually performed during an EGD. A dilating (stretching) procedure can also be done if a tumor is obstructing

Upper endoscopy

Upper endoscopy allows your doctor to see the inner wall of your stomach and esophagus. If ultrasound is used, your doctor will be able to see the deeper wall layers and nearby organs.

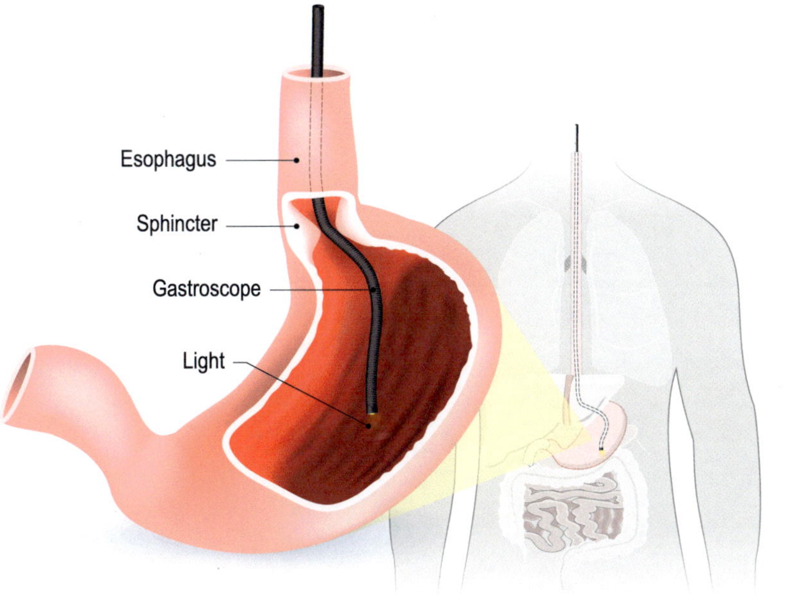

the esophagus. After the endoscopy, your throat may feel sore, and you may feel some swelling.

Bronchoscopy

During a bronchoscopy, a device is inserted through the nose or mouth to examine the inside of your airway, including the trachea and bronchi. Bronchoscopy may be used to detect cancer from the esophagus or to perform some treatment procedures.

Laparoscopy

Laparoscopy (key-hole surgery or minimally invasive surgery) is a surgical procedure that inserts a camera and various instruments (laparoscope) through small cuts (ports) in the abdomen. During the procedure, a tool can take tissue samples or remove tumors. Laparoscopy is done under general anesthesia. This is a loss of feeling and a complete loss of awareness that feels like a very deep sleep.

Biopsy

A biopsy removes a sample of tissue or fluid during an upper endoscopy. Several samples may be taken from the tumor, wall of your esophagus or stomach, and lymph nodes. The samples will be sent to a pathologist, an expert in examining cells under a microscope to find disease.

Other types of biopsies may include:

- **Fine-needle aspiration (FNA) or core biopsy (CB)** uses needles of different sizes to remove a sample of tissue or fluid. An endoscopic ultrasound (EUS) may guide the FNA for diagnosis.
- **Brushings or washings** involve removing tumor or cell samples with a small brush at the end of an endoscope.
- **Liquid biopsy** uses a sample of blood for testing.

Biopsy of metastases

A metastasis is the spread of cancer to an area of the body such as the lung, liver, kidney, bone, or distant lymph nodes. A biopsy of the metastasis may be needed to confirm the presence of cancer. If there is more than one metastasis, each site may be biopsied. The type of biopsy used depends on the location of the suspected metastases and other factors.

Biomarker testing

A sample from a biopsy of your tumor may be tested to look for specific DNA (deoxyribonucleic acid) mutations (abnormal changes), protein levels, or other molecular features. It is sometimes called molecular testing or tumor profiling. Biomarker testing includes tests of genes or their products (proteins). It identifies the presence or absence of mutations and certain proteins that might guide prognosis or treatment. Proteins are written like this: NTRK. Genes are written in italics like this: *NTRK*. Your care team will recommend the best types of biomarker testing for you.

Immunohistochemistry (IHC), fluorescence in situ hybridization (FISH), polymerase chain reaction (PCR), or next-generation sequencing (NGS) are types of tests used to look for biomarkers.

Testing for HER2 status, microsatellite instability (MSI) status, programmed death ligand 1 (PD-L1) expression, tumor mutational burden, neurotrophic tropomyosinrelated kinase (*NTRK*), and rearranged during transfection (*RET*) gene fusions as well as *BRAF* V600E (gene that encodes a protein B-raf) mutation are important for the treatment and management of advanced esophageal cancer.

Tumor mutation testing

Tumor mutation testing or tumor genomic aberration testing uses a sample of your tumor or blood to see if the cancer cells have any specific DNA mutations. This information may be used to guide certain drug choices. This is a different type of DNA testing than the genetic testing for mutations you may have inherited from your biological parents. In tumor mutation testing, only the tumor is tested and not the rest of your body. Many mutations such as *NTRK* gene fusions can be targeted with specific therapies.

> **“From the moment you get a cancer diagnosis, you are thrust into a world of new terms, many of them vital to understanding what is happening to you. It’s important to understand what biomarkers are and even how these biomarkers can affect treatments.”**

HER2

Human epidermal growth factor receptor 2 (HER2) is a protein involved in normal cell growth. It is found on the surface of all cells. When amounts are high, it causes cells to grow and divide. This is called HER2 positive (HER2+), overexpression, or amplification.

There might be higher amounts of HER2 in your esophageal cancer. A sample of your tumor might be tested for HER2. If your tumor makes too much HER2, you might receive a targeted therapy called trastuzumab (Herceptin) or a biosimilar, or trastuzumab deruxtecan (Enhertu). A biosimilar is an almost identical version of trastuzumab made by another company. It is used in the exact same way and at the same dose as trastuzumab.

MSI-H/dMMR

Microsatellites are short, repeated strings of DNA that are fixed by mismatch repair (MMR) proteins. Some cancers prevent these errors from being fixed. This is called microsatellite instability (MSI) or deficient mismatch repair (dMMR). When cancer cells have more than a normal number of microsatellites, it is called microsatellite instability-high (MSI-H). This is often due to dMMR genes.

Tumor mutational burden

When there are 10 or more mutations per million base pairs of tumor DNA, it is called tumor mutational burden-high (TMB-H). TMB-H can be used to help predict response to cancer treatment using immune checkpoint inhibitors that target the proteins called programmed death protein 1 (PD-1) and programmed death-ligand 1 (PD-L1).

PD-L1

Programmed death-ligand 1 (PD-L1) is an immune protein. If this protein is expressed on the surface of cancer cells, it can cause your immune cells to ignore the cancer and suppress the anti-tumor immune response. If your cancer expresses the PD-L1 protein, you might have treatment that combines chemotherapy and checkpoint inhibitor therapy. This is designed to activate your immune system to better fight off the cancer cells.

If you smoke or vape, seek help to quit

A history of smoking or vaping nicotine increases your chances of developing lung and other cancers. Smoking and vaping can limit how well cancer treatment works and prevents wound healing. It also greatly increases your chances of having side effects during and after surgery. Cannabis use might also affect the amount of anesthesia used during surgery.

Nicotine is the chemical in tobacco that makes you want to keep smoking and vaping. Nicotine withdrawal is challenging for most people who smoke or vape. The stress of having cancer may make it even harder to quit. If you smoke or vape, ask your care team about counseling and medicines to help you quit.

For online support, try these websites:

- SmokeFree.gov
- BeTobaccoFree.gov
- CDC.gov/tobacco

NTRK gene fusions

In a tumor with an *NTRK* gene fusion, a piece of the *NTRK* gene and a piece of another gene fuse or join. This activates the *NTRK* gene in a way that causes uncontrolled cell growth. Larotrectinib (Vitrakvi) and entrectinib (Rozlytrek) might be used to target tumors with a *NTRK* gene fusion.

RET gene fusions

Rearranged during transfection (*RET*) gene mutation is related to cell growth (proliferation). Selpercatinib (Retevmo) might be used for esophageal cancer with a *RET* gene fusion.

BRAF V600E

Mutations in the *BRAF* gene can cause normal cells to become cancerous. Dabrafenib (Tafinlar) and trametinib (Mekinist) might be used for tumors with *BRAF* V600E mutations.

FISH

Fluorescence in situ hybridization (FISH) is a lab testing method that involves special dyes called probes that attach to pieces of DNA, the genetic material in a person's cells. This can tell how many copies of a gene are present in the cell.

Immunohistochemistry

Immunohistochemistry (IHC) is a staining process that involves using a chemical marker to detect cell proteins such as HER2 and PD-L1. The cells are then studied using a microscope.

Next-generation sequencing

Next-generation sequencing (NGS) is a high-throughput method used to determine a portion of a person's DNA sequence. This method would only be used if enough tumor tissue remains after other biomarker testing has been completed.

PCR

A polymerase chain reaction (PCR) is a lab process that can make millions or billions of copies of your DNA (genetic information). PCR is very sensitive. It can find 1 abnormal cell among more than 100,000 normal cells. These copies called PCR product might be used for NGS.

Liquid biopsy

Some mutations can be found by testing circulating tumor DNA (ctDNA) in the blood. In a liquid biopsy, a sample of blood is taken to look for cancer cells or for pieces of DNA from tumor cells. This is similar to NGS but uses a blood sample rather than a tissue sample.

Those who have metastatic or advanced esophageal cancer and are unable to undergo a traditional biopsy might have a liquid biopsy. Sometimes testing can quickly use up a tumor sample and a liquid biopsy might be an option in this case. The number of genes assessed by liquid biopsy is less than in tisssue-based NGS.

Genetic risk testing

Genetic risk testing is done using blood or saliva (spitting into a cup). The goal is to look for gene mutations inherited from your genetic parents called germline mutations. Some mutations can put you at risk for more than one type of cancer. You can pass these genes on to your children. Also, family members might carry these mutations. Tell your doctor if there is a family history of cancer. Depending on your family history or other features of your cancer, your health care provider might refer you for hereditary genetic testing to learn more about your cancer. A genetic counselor will speak to you about the results.

Hereditary syndromes

Certain genetic (inherited) syndromes may put someone at risk for developing esophageal cancer. A syndrome is a group of signs or symptoms that occur together and suggest the presence of or risk for a disease.

A genetic risk assessment will identify if you carry a cancer risk and if you may benefit from genetic testing, additional screening, or preventive interventions. Depending on the genetic risk assessment, you might undergo genetic testing and genetic counseling.

Hereditary syndromes most closely related to esophageal and EGJ cancers include:

- Esophageal cancer, tylosis with non-epidermolytic palmoplantar keratoderma (PPK), and Howel-Evans syndrome
- Familial Barrett esophagus (FBE)
- Bloom syndrome (BS)
- Fanconi anemia (FA)

Performance status

Performance status (PS) is a person's general level of fitness and ability to perform daily tasks. Your state of general health will be rated using a PS scale called Eastern Cooperative Oncology Group (ECOG) or the Karnofsky Performance Status (KPS). PS is one factor taken into consideration when choosing a treatment plan. In general, a lower PS means that it will be harder for you to tolerate cancer drugs. Your preferences about treatment are always important.

ECOG PS

The ECOG PS scores range from 0 to 5.

- PS 0 means the person is fully active.
- PS 1 means the person is still able to perform light to moderate activity, but with some limitations.
- PS 2 means the person is limited to the chair or bed less than half of the day and still able to care for self.
- PS 3 means the person is limited to the chair or bed more than half of the day.
- PS 4 means the person is totally confined to the bed or chair and completely unable to care for self.
- PS 5 means the person is not alive.

In esophageal cancer, PS might be referred to as good or poor. Good PS is usually PS 0 or PS 1.

Karnofsky PS

The KPS score ranges from 0 to 100.

- 10 to 40 means you cannot care for yourself.
- 50 to 70 means you cannot work and need some help to take care of yourself.
- 80 to 100 means you can carry out daily tasks.

We want your feedback!

Our goal is to provide helpful and easy-to-understand information on cancer.

Take our survey to let us know what we got right and what we could do better.

NCCN.org/patients/feedback

Performance status

Performance status (PS) is a person's ability to perform daily tasks.

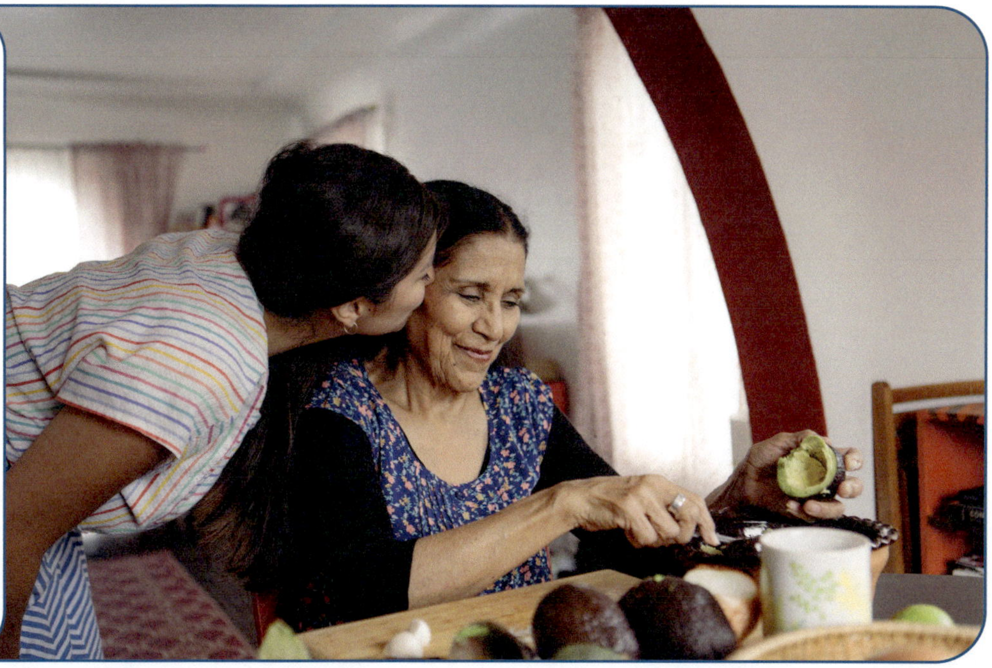

Key points

- Tests are used to find cancer, plan treatment, and check how well treatment is working.
- Blood tests check for signs of disease and how well organs are working.
- Imaging tests take pictures of the inside of your body. Images can be made with scanning machines or scoping tools.
- A biopsy removes a sample of tissue or fluid during an endoscopy.
- A sample of blood may be used to assess tumor genetics.
- A sample from a biopsy of your tumor may be tested to look for specific DNA mutations, protein expression levels, or other molecular features. Some mutations and proteins can be targeted with specific therapies.
- Genetic risk testing might be done to look for gene mutations inherited from your birth parents called germline mutations.

“

Knowing there is treatment available gave me hope at diagnosis and for the future.”

3

Staging

Cancer staging is used to make treatment decisions. It describes the size and location (or extent) of the tumor, if the tumor has grown through the layers of the esophagus wall, and if cancer has spread to lymph nodes, organs, or other parts of the body. This chapter explains esophageal cancer stages.

Siewert types

Siewert types are helpful in telling the difference between a stomach and esophageal cancer. A Siewert type describes tumors located in the area of the esophagus near the stomach. This area is called the esophagogastric junction (EGJ) and the cardia (the opening where the esophagus meets the stomach). The EGJ is found just beneath the diaphragm.

EGJ tumors located within 2 cm of the stomach (Siewert Types I and II) are staged as esophageal adenocarcinoma. Cancers whose center is more than 2 cm below the EGJ, even if the EGJ is involved, will be staged using the stomach cancer tumor, node, metastasis (TNM) and stage groups.

- **Siewert Type I** – The tumor center is located within 1 to 5 cm above the EGJ and cardia.
- **Siewert Type II** – The tumor center is located within 1 cm above and 2 cm below the EGJ.
- **Siewert Type III** – The tumor center is located between 2 to 5 cm below the

Siewert types

A Siewert type describes tumors located in the area of esophagus near the stomach. Siewert types I and II are treated as esophageal cancer. Siewert type III is treated as stomach cancer. There are some exceptions.

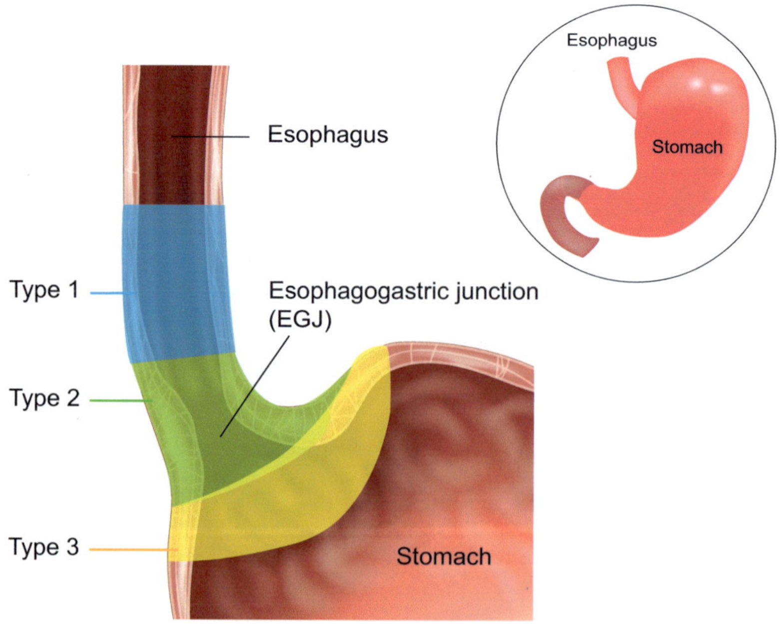

EGJ, which infiltrates the EGJ and the lower esophagus from below.

Siewert Type III tumors are considered and treated as stomach (gastric) cancers. For more information, see *NCCN Guidelines for Patients: Stomach Cancer*, available at NCCN.org/patientguidelines and on the NCCN Patient Guides for Cancer app.

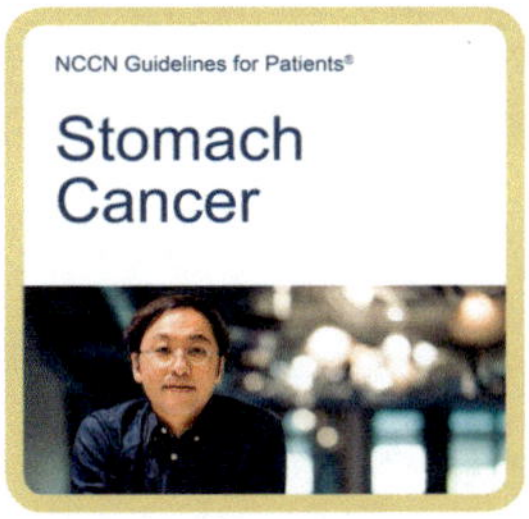

Staging

Esophageal cancer staging is often done twice: before any treatment and after surgery.

- **Clinical stage (c)** is the rating given before any treatment. It is based on a physical exam, biopsy, and imaging tests. An example might look like cN2 or cM1.
- **Pathologic stage (p)** or surgical stage is determined by examining tissue removed during surgery. An example might be pN2. If you are given drug therapy before surgery (neoadjuvant), then the stage might use a y before it and look like ypT3.

A cancer stage is a way to describe the extent of the cancer at the time you are first diagnosed. The American Joint Committee on Cancer (AJCC) created a staging system to determine how much cancer is in your body, where it is located, and what subtype you have. AJCC is just one type of staging system.

Staging is based on a combination of information to reach a final numbered stage.

Often, not all information is available at the initial evaluation. More information can be gathered as treatment begins. Doctors may explain your cancer stage in different ways than described next.

TNM scores

The tumor, node, metastasis (TNM) system is used to stage esophageal cancer. In this system, the letters T, N, and M describe different areas of cancer growth. Based on imaging and pathology results, a score or number is assigned to each letter. The higher the number, the larger the tumor or the more the cancer has spread to lymph nodes or other organs. These scores will be combined to assign the cancer a stage. A TNM example might look like this: T1N0M0 or T1, N0, M0.

The TNM letters represent the following:

- **T (tumor)** – Depth and spread of the main (primary) tumor in the wall of esophagus
- **N (node)** – If cancer has spread to nearby (regional) lymph nodes
- **M (metastasis)** – If cancer has spread to distant parts of the body or metastasized

A specific diagnosis of esophageal squamous cell carcinoma (SCC) or adenocarcinoma is needed for staging and treatment purposes. Mixed adenosquamous carcinomas and carcinomas are staged using the TNM system for SCC.

Grade

Grade describes how abnormal the tumor cells look under a microscope (called histology). Higher-grade cancers tend to grow and spread faster than lower-grade cancers. GX means the grade can't be determined, followed by G1, G2, and G3. Well differentiated (G1) means the cancer cells look similar to normal cells.

Poorly differentiated (G3) means the cancer cells look very different compared to normal cells. G3 is the highest grade for esophageal cancers.

- **GX** – Grade cannot be determined
- **G1** – Well differentiated
- **G2** – Moderately differentiated
- **G3** – Poorly differentiated or undifferentiated

Numbered stages

Numbered stages are based on TNM scores. Stages range from stage 1 to stage 4, with 4 being the most advanced. They might be written as stage I, stage II, stage III, and stage IV.

Other terms might be used instead of numbered cancer stages. This book will use the following terms to describe esophageal cancer:

- **Resectable** – Tumor can be removed completely with surgery.
- **Unresectable** – Tumor cannot be removed with surgery. It might involve nearby veins and arteries making it unsafe to remove.
- **Locoregional or locally advanced** – Tumor might be any size and could be in any layer of the esophagus. Cancer might

Regional lymph nodes

A tumor can be found anywhere in the esophagus. Cancer may be found in lymph nodes along the esophagus.

https://commons.wikimedia.org/wiki/File:Diagram_showing_oesophageal_cancer_in_the_lymph_nodes_(N_staging)_CRUK_174.svg

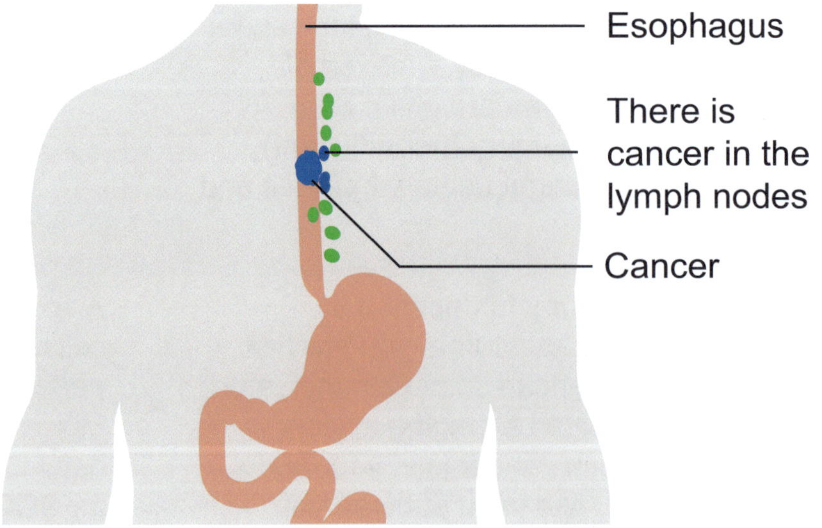

be in nearby lymph nodes, organs, and tissues.

- **Metastatic** – Cancer has spread to other parts of the body, including distant lymph nodes. The most common metastatic sites are the liver, distant lymph nodes, lung, bone, and brain.

T = Tumor

A tumor can grow through the layers of the esophagus wall and into nearby structures.

- **Tis** – High-grade dysplasia (HGD) is cancer that has not grown beyond the epithelium.
- **T1** – Tumor invades the lamina propria, muscularis mucosa, or submucosa.
  - **T1a** – Tumor invades the lamina propria or muscularis mucosa.
  - **T1b** – Tumor invades the submucosa.
- **T2** – Tumor invades the muscle layer called muscularis propria.
- **T3** – Tumor invades the adventitia.
- **T4** – Tumor has grown all the way through the wall of the esophagus into nearby structures.
  - **T4a** – Tumor has grown into nearby structures, such as the pleura, pericardium, azygos vein, diaphragm, or peritoneum. The pleura covers the lungs and lines the interior wall of the chest cavity. The pericardium is the sac that surrounds the heart. The azygos vein is a blood vessel that carries blood from the back walls of the chest and abdomen to the heart. The peritoneum lines the abdominal wall and covers most of the organs in the abdomen.
  - **T4b** – Tumor has grown into nearby structures, such as the aorta, spinal column, heart, or airway (trachea).

Tis and T1 tumors are often considered early-stage cancer. Esophageal cancers are rarely found this early.

N = Regional lymph node

There are hundreds of lymph nodes throughout your body. They work as filters to help fight infection and remove harmful things from your body. Regional lymph nodes are found near the esophagus. Cancer found in a lymph node is called a lymph node metastasis. This is different than a distant metastasis, which is found farther from the main tumor in the esophagus.

Lymph, a clear fluid containing cells that help fight infections and other diseases, drains through channels from the wall of the esophagus into lymphatic vessels in the mucosa and submucosa. From here, lymph drains into lymph nodes outside and along the esophagus. These lymph nodes drain into the thoracic duct. It is possible for cancer cells to travel through lymph to other parts of the body.

Since the lymphatic network is concentrated in the submucosa, lymph node metastases can be found in early-stage cancers.

Lymph nodes must be removed to confirm cancer. The removal of many lymph nodes is called lymph node dissection (lymphadenectomy). It might be referred to as a nodal dissection. At least 15 lymph nodes should be removed in curative surgery when the esophageal tumor is also removed.

- **N0** – No cancer is found in nearby lymph nodes.
- **N1** – 1 or 2 nearby nodes have cancer.
- **N2** – 3 to 6 nearby nodes have cancer.
- **N3** – 7 or more nearby lymph nodes have cancer.

M = Metastasis

Cancer that has spread to distant parts of the body is shown as M1. The most common metastatic sites are the liver, distant lymph nodes, and lung.

Clinical stage

The clinical (before surgery) stage is based on the endoscopic ultrasound (EUS) and other imaging or biopsy results. These tests are done before any treatment as part of an initial diagnosis.

Clinical stages for esophageal squamous cell carcinomas can be found in **Guide 2**.

Clinical stages for esophageal adenocarcinomas can be found in **Guide 3.**

Guide 2
Squamous cell carcinoma stages: Clinical (cTNM)

Stage 0	• Tis, N0, M0
Stage 1	• T1, N0 or N1, M0
Stage 2	• T2, N0 or N1, M0 • T3, N0, M0
Stage 3	• T3, N1, M0 • T1 to T3, N2, M0
Stage 4A	• T4, N0 to N2, M0 • Any T, N3, M0
Stage 4B	• Any T, Any N1, M1

Guide 3
Adenocarcinoma stages: Clinical (cTNM)

Stage 0	• Tis, N0, M0
Stage 1	• T1, N0, M0
Stage 2A	• T1, N1, M0
Stage 2B	• T2, N0, M0
Stage 3	• T2, N1, M0 • T3, N0 to N1, M0 • T4a, N0 to N1, M0
Stage 4A	• T1 to T4a, N2, M0 • T4b, N0 to N2, M0 • Any T, N3, M0
Stage 4B	• Any T, Any N, M1

Pathologic stage

The pathologic (after surgery) stage is based on information gained after surgery that's aim was to remove part or all of the esophagus and nearby lymph nodes. This gives a more accurate picture of how far the cancer has spread and is used to determine your treatment options after surgery. The removal of tumor tissue and nearby lymph nodes is an important part of pathologic staging and treatment of the cancer.

Pathologic stages for esophageal squamous cell carcinomas can be found in **Guide 4**.

Guide 4
Squamous cell carcinoma stages: Pathologic (pTNM) and grade (G)

Stage 0	• Tis, N0, M0, any location
Stage 1A	• T1a, N0, M0, GX or G1, any location
Stage 1B	• T1a, N0, M0, G2 or G3, any location • T1b, N0, M0, G1 to G3, any location • T1b, N0, M0, GX, any location • T2, N0, M0, G1, any location
Stage 2A	• T2, N0, M0, G2 or G3, any location • T2, N0, M0, GX, any location • T3, N0, M0, G1 to G3, lower esophagus • T3, N0, M0, G1, upper or middle esophagus
Stage 2B	• T3, N0, M0, G2 or G3, upper or middle esophagus • T3, N0, M0, GX, lower or upper or middle esophagus • T3, N0, M0, any grade, location unknown • T1, N1, M0, any grade, any location
Stage 3A	• T1, N2, M0, any grade, any location • T2, N1, M0, any grade, any location
Stage 3B	• T2, N2, M0, any grade, any location • T3, N1 or N2, M0, any grade, any location • T4b, N0 or N1, M0, any grade, any location
Stage 4A	• T4a, N2, M0, any grade, any location • T4b, N0 or N1 or N2, M0, any grade, any location • Any T, N3, M0, any grade, any location
Stage 4B	• Any T, any N, M1, any grade, any location

Pathologic stages for esophageal adenocarcinomas can be found in **Guide 5**.

Guide 5
Adenocarcinoma stages: Pathologic (pTNM) and grade (G)

Stage 0	• Tis, N0, M0
Stage 1A	• T1a, N0, M0, GX or G1
Stage 1B	• T1a, N0, M0, G2 • T1b, N0, M0, GX or G1 or G2
Stage 1C	• T1, N0, M0, G3 • T2, N0, M0, G1 or G2
Stage 2A	• T2, N0, M0, GX or G3
Stage 2B	• T1, N1, M0, any grade • T3, N0, M0, any grade
Stage 3A	• T1, N2, M0, any grade • T2, N1, M0, any grade
Stage 3B	• T2, N2, M0, any grade • T3, N1 or N2, M0, any grade • T4b, N0 or N1, M0, any grade
Stage 4A	• T4a, N2, M0, any grade • T4b, N0 or N1 or N2, M0, any grade • Any T, N3, M0, any grade
Stage 4B	• Any T, Any N, M1, any grade

Key points

- Staging is used to make treatment decisions. Staging describes how much cancer is in your body and where it is located.
- The tumor, node, metastasis (TNM) system is used to stage esophageal cancer.
- Esophageal cancer staging is often done twice: before and after surgery.
- The clinical stage (c) of esophageal cancer is based on the results of testing done before endoscopic resection or surgery. It is written as cTNM.
- The pathologic stage (p) of esophageal cancer is based on the examination of the tumor removed by endoscopic resection or surgery. It is written as pTNM.
- Staging information after treatment and surgery is written as ypTNM.
- Cancer that has spread to distant parts of the body is metastatic cancer.

"It's OK to have bad days but don't let yourself stay there. A positive attitude goes a long way."

4

Treating esophageal cancer

There is more than one treatment for esophageal cancer. This chapter describes treatment options and what to expect. Together, you and your doctor will choose a treatment plan that is best for you.

Need help paying for medicine or treatment?

Ask your care team what options are available.

Care team

Those with esophageal cancer should seek treatment at experienced cancer centers.

Treating esophageal cancer takes a team approach. Treatment decisions should involve a multidisciplinary team (MDT). An MDT is a team of doctors, health care workers, and social care professionals from different professional backgrounds who have knowledge (expertise) and experience with your type of cancer. This team is united in the planning and implementing of your treatment. Ask who will coordinate your care.

Some members of your care team will be with you throughout cancer treatment, while others will only be there for parts of it. Get to know your care team and help them get to know you.

Your cancer care is not just about physical and mental health but also financial health. You might feel shy asking about how your care might affect you financially. But it's important to find out all you can about the costs. Your care team understands and will want to answer your questions, so feel free to ask them. Depending on your diagnosis, your team might include the following specialists:

- **A gastroenterologist** is an expert in diseases of the digestive tract.
- **A surgical oncologist** performs operations to remove cancer, including the esophagus.
- **A thoracic surgical oncologist** performs operations to remove organs that involve the chest, including the esophagus.
- **A medical oncologist** treats cancer using systemic (drug) therapy.
- **A radiation oncologist** prescribes and plans radiation therapy to treat cancer.
- **Oncology nurses** provide your hands-on care, like giving systemic therapy, managing your care, answering questions, and helping you cope with side effects.
- **Oncology pharmacists** are experts in knowing how to use medicines to treat cancer and to manage symptoms and side effects.
- **Palliative care specialists** concentrate on preventing and alleviating suffering and improving quality of life.

- **Nutritionists and dietitians** can provide guidance on what foods are most suitable for your condition.
- **Psychologists and psychiatrists** are mental health experts who can help manage issues such as depression, anxiety, or other mental health conditions that can affect how you feel.
- **Social workers** help people solve and cope with problems in their everyday lives. Clinical social workers also diagnose and treat mental, behavioral, and emotional issues. The anxiety a person feels when diagnosed with cancer might be managed by a social worker in some cancer centers. They, or other designated professionals, can help navigate the complexities of financial and insurance stresses.
- **Spiritual care specialists** identify and support those with spiritual distress or unmet spiritual needs.
- **Smoking cessation specialists** can provide medication and counseling for those who would like to stop using tobacco or nicotine products.
- **A research team** helps to collect research data if you are in a clinical trial. Clinical trials help bring new therapies to patients and advance the treatment for everyone. Consider asking your care team about access to clinical trials.

Many cancer centers and hospitals offer several free or low-cost services and programs to help you navigate your treatment and help you connect with other people with cancer. Feel free to find out more by asking your care team about them.

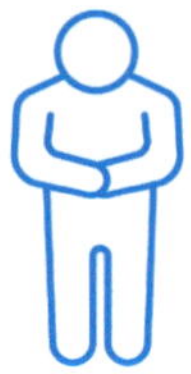

You know your body better than anyone

Help your care team understand:

- ✓ How you feel
- ✓ What you need
- ✓ What is working and what is not

Keep a list of names and contact information for each member of your team. This will make it easier for you and anyone involved in your care to know whom to contact with questions or concerns.

Get to know your care team and help them get to know you.

Endoscopic therapy

Some treatments use a thin, tube-shaped tool called an endoscope that is inserted into the body to take pictures. One end of the scope has a small light and camera lens to see inside your body. The image is displayed on a television monitor. This will help guide your doctor for a biopsy, treatment, or other tasks. An endoscope is often guided into the body through the mouth.

The goal of endoscopic therapy is to remove or destroy early-stage disease and Barrett esophagus (BE). Endoscopic resection (ER) with or without ablation is preferred for early-stage cancer.

Endoscopic resection is a minimally invasive procedure that uses an endoscope to remove precancerous and cancerous areas of the esophagus.

Endoscopic resection

For those with early-stage (T1a or T1b) esophageal cancer or BE, endoscopic mucosal resection (EMR) or endoscopic submucosal dissection (ESD) is essential for accurate staging and diagnosis.

Early-stage esophageal cancer has not grown beyond the first layer (mucosa) of the esophagus wall. The tumor is often very small (2 centimeters or less) and is not in any lymph nodes.

Endoscopic mucosal resection

Endoscopic mucosal resection (EMR) is a procedure to remove pre-cancerous, early-stage cancer or other abnormal tissues (lesions) from the esophagus wall. During EMR, the endoscope is passed down your throat to reach the lesion or tumor in your esophagus. The lesion can be removed through suction or by cutting it away. Talk to your doctor to learn more.

Endoscopic submucosal dissection

Endoscopic submucosal dissection (ESD) uses an endoscope to locate the tumor in the esophagus wall. A tool is inserted through the endoscope that injects fluid between the tumor and layer of the esophageal wall. Then a tool lifts and cuts away the tumor from the esophageal wall.

Ablation

Ablation uses extreme cold or extreme heat, radio waves, microwaves, or chemicals to destroy cancer cells. It can destroy small tumors and metastases with little harm to nearby tissue. You might have multiple treatments to destroy the tumor or metastasis. Ablation might be used if you are not healthy enough for surgery.

There are many types of ablation used to destroy cancer cells. Those most commonly used to treat an esophageal tumor include:

- **Cryotherapy or cryosurgery** kills cancer cells by freezing them with a very cold substance.
- **Radiofrequency ablation (RFA)** kills cancer cells by heating them with high-energy radio waves.
- **Photodynamic therapy (PTD)** uses drugs that become active when exposed to light. These activated drugs may kill cancer cells.

Surgery and endoscopic procedures are best performed by experienced surgeons and endoscopists in high-volume centers for esophageal cancer. High volume means performing dozens of procedures per year.

Surgery

Surgery is an operation or procedure to remove cancer from the body. Often, surgery is the main or primary treatment to remove the cancer from the esophagus. This is only one part of a treatment plan. Surgery can also provide supportive care by easing pain or discomfort. This is called palliative surgery.

When preparing for surgery, seek the opinion of an experienced surgeon. The surgeon should be an expert in performing your type of surgery. Surgery for esophageal cancer should be done at a high-volume center that does at least 15 to 20 esophageal surgeries each year (as well as having on staff multidisciplinary teams and dedicated thoracic surgical, medical, and radiation oncologists). Hospitals that perform many surgeries often have better results. You can ask for a referral to a hospital or cancer center that has experience in treating your type of cancer.

The removal of the cancer through surgery can be accomplished in different ways depending on the specific circumstances, such as the size and location of the tumor, and if there is cancer in any surrounding organs and tissues. Surgery is based on the safest and best way to remove the cancer.

Open surgery

Open surgery may include incisions in the chest (thoracotomy), abdomen (laparotomy), or neck. These larger incisions let your doctor directly view and access the tumor in your esophagus to remove it. Open surgery may take several hours or longer. After the surgery, you will need to stay in the hospital for several days or longer to recover.

Minimally invasive surgery

Minimally invasive surgery (key-hole surgery) uses several small incisions. Small tools are inserted through each incision to perform the surgery. One of the tools, called a videoscope, is a long tube with a video camera at the end. The camera lets your doctor see your esophagus and other tissues inside your chest and abdomen. Other tools are used to remove the tumor. Minimally invasive surgery, also called thoracoscopic and laparoscopic surgery, can also be done using robotic arms to control the surgical tools. This is called robot-assisted or robotic surgery.

Tumor resection

Imaging tests will be ordered to see if your cancer is resectable (can be removed completely by surgery) or unresectable (cannot be removed completely by surgery). Sometimes, imaging and scoping tests cannot clearly show one way or the other.

Goal of surgery

The goal of surgery (tumor resection) is to remove all of the cancer. To do so, the tumor is removed along with some normal-looking tissue around its edge called the surgical margin. The surgical margin may look normal, but cancerous cells may be found when viewed under a microscope by a pathologist. A clear or negative margin (R0) is when no cancer cells are found in the tissue around the edge of the tumor. In a positive margin, cancer cells are found in normal-looking tissue around the tumor.

You may receive treatment before surgery called neoadjuvant, induction, or preoperative therapy. Neoadjuvant therapy will help reduce the size of the tumor and the amount of cancer in the body.

Surgical margins

The goal of surgery is a cancer-free surgical margin with reasonable functional outcome. This is your ability to perform daily tasks of living. After surgery, you may receive treatment such as radiation, chemoradiation, or systemic therapy to kill any remaining cancer cells.

- **In a clear or negative margin (R0),** no cancerous cells are found in the tissue around the edge of the tumor.
- **In an R1 positive margin,** the surgeon removes all the visible tumor, but the microscopic edges are still positive for tumor cells. Despite best efforts, this can happen.
- **In an R2 positive margin,** the surgeon is unable to remove all the visible tumor or there is metastatic disease (M1).

A negative margin (R0) is the best result. Your surgeon will look carefully for cancer not only along the surgical margin, but in other nearby areas. An intraoperative pathology consultation is often used by surgeons. This includes inspecting the resected esophageal tissue for cancer location and distance to margins, examining by microscope frozen sections of the margins, and examining by microscope for possible metastasis such as in the liver or abdomen. Intraoperative pathology consultation serves an important role in guiding the surgery.

Despite best efforts, it is not always possible to find all of the cancer. Sometimes, surgeons can't safely remove the tumor with a cancer-free margin.

You might have more than one surgery. You might also have a wound drain to prevent fluid from collecting in the body after surgery. These drains are usually removed a few days after surgery.

Esophagectomy

An esophagectomy removes part, most, or all of the esophagus. An esophagectomy is a big operation, even when it uses a minimally invasive approach. The surgery crosses two or three body cavities—abdomen, chest, and neck—and usually takes 4 to 6 hours. Eating a healthy diet and exercising before surgery is important. When you are in your best possible physical condition before surgery, it is more likely that you will experience a quicker and easier recovery after surgery.

Types of esophagectomy include:

- **A transhiatal esophagectomy (THE)** is performed through creating an opening on the neck and abdomen. Typically, the stomach is joined to the esophagus in the neck.
- **A transthoracic esophagectomy (TTE)** is performed through creating an opening on the abdomen and the chest, and occasionally in the neck as well. The stomach may be joined to the esophagus in the chest or in the neck, depending on the location of the tumor.

Minimally invasive laparoscopic and thoracoscopic or robotic surgical approaches may be incorporated in esophagectomy.

Before and after an esophagectomy

These images show before and after an esophagectomy. In this case, a large portion of the esophagus has been removed. The stomach has been pulled up and joined with the esophagus. Sometimes, instead of the stomach, a piece of the small intestine or colon is used to replace the missing part of the esophagus.

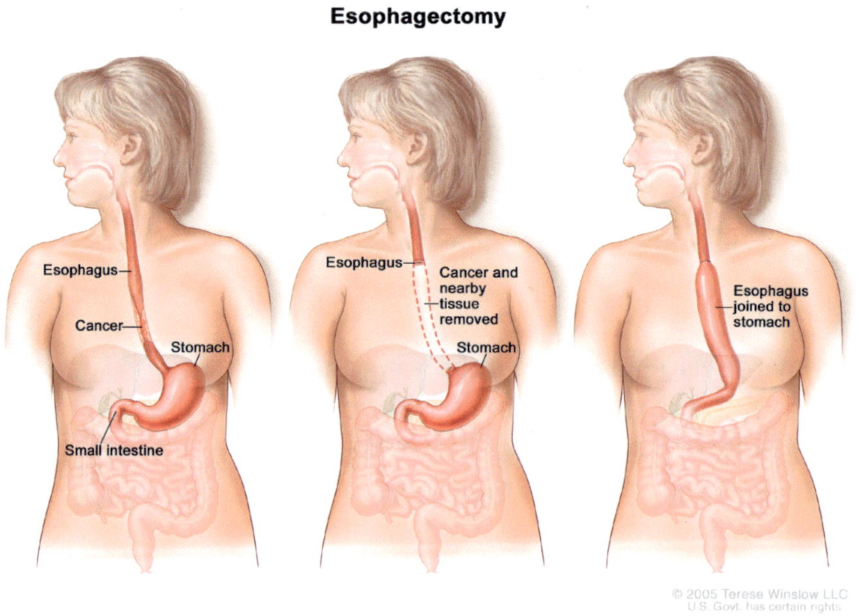

Reconstruction conduits

A conduit is a tube-shaped tissue, such as the stomach, the colon, or small intestine, used to replace or reconstruct the part of the esophagus removed during an esophagectomy. A stomach (gastric) conduit is preferred and is the most commonly used conduit for esophageal reconstruction. The stomach is a large, durable organ with abundant blood supply.

The type of esophageal resection is dictated by the location of the tumor, the available choices for conduit, and the surgeon's experience and preference, as well as your preference.

Other procedures

Esophagogastrectomy

In an esophagogastrectomy, the top part of the stomach and distal part of the esophagus are removed. A nutritionist or dietician provides guidance on what foods are most suitable for you before and after this surgery.

Lymph node dissection

The removal of lymph nodes or groups of lymph nodes is called lymph node or nodal dissection. It might be referred to as a lymphadenectomy. At least 15 regional nodes should be removed and tested for cancer.

G-tube

A gastrostomy tube (G-tube) is a soft, plastic tube placed through the skin of the abdomen directly into the stomach. It allows air and fluid to leave the stomach and can be used to give medicines and fluids, including liquid food. Giving food through a gastrostomy tube is a type of enteral nutrition. It is also called a percutaneous endoscopic gastrostomy (PEG) tube.

J-tube

A jejunostomy tube (J-tube) is a soft, plastic tube placed through the skin of the abdomen into the midsection of the small intestine. The tube delivers food and medicine until you are healthy enough to eat by mouth.

Systemic therapy

Systemic therapy works throughout the body. Types include chemotherapy, targeted therapy, and immunotherapy. Systemic therapy might be used alone or with other therapies. Goals and side effects of systemic therapy should be discussed with your care team before starting treatment. Having a better idea of what to expect can help inform your wishes about treatment.

- **Neoadjuvant or preoperative therapy** is systemic therapy or chemoradiation given before surgery.
- **Perioperative therapy** is systemic therapy given before and after surgery.
- **Adjuvant or postoperative therapy** is systemic therapy or radiation therapy given after surgery.
- **Palliative therapy** is systemic therapy given for advanced disease.

Chemotherapy

Chemotherapy kills fast-growing cells throughout the body, including cancer cells and some normal cells. When chemotherapies are combined, it is called multi-agent or combination chemotherapy. Chemotherapy might be used before and after surgery. It might be used with radiation (called chemoradiation).

Some examples of chemotherapies include:

- Capecitabine (Xeloda)
- Carboplatin
- Cisplatin
- Docetaxel (Taxotere)
- Fluorouracil
- Irinotecan (Camptosar)
- Oxaliplatin (Eloxatin)
- Paclitaxel (Taxol)

Chemoradiation

Treatment that combines chemotherapy with radiation therapy is called chemoradiation. Chemotherapy may improve how well radiation works, and that is why they are sometimes used together. Chemoradiation may be used to control symptoms caused by a tumor, to shrink the tumor before surgery, to prevent the return of cancer after surgery, or as the primary (main) treatment for the tumor.

Warnings about supplements and drug interactions

You might be asked to stop taking or avoid certain herbal supplements when on a systemic therapy. Some supplements can affect the ability of a drug to do its job. This is called a drug interaction.

It is critical to speak with your care team about any supplements you may be taking. Some examples include:

- Turmeric
- Ginkgo biloba
- Green tea extract
- St. John's Wort
- Antioxidants

Certain medicines can also affect the ability of a drug to do its job. Antacids, heart or blood pressure medicine, and antidepressants are just some of the medicines that might interact with a systemic therapy or supportive care medicines given during systemic therapy. Therefore, it is very important to tell your care team about any medicines, vitamins, over-the-counter (OTC) drugs, herbals, or supplements you are taking.

Bring a list with you to every visit.

Immunotherapy

Immunotherapy can be given alone or with other types of treatment. Immunotherapy is a systemic treatment that tries to reactivate your own immune system against tumor cells. The immune system has many on and off switches. Tumors take advantage of off switches. Some immunotherapy examples are nivolumab (Opdivo), pembrolizumab (Keytruda), tislelizumab-jsgr (Tevimbra), and dostarlimab-gxly (Jemperli).

More information on checkpoint inhibitors and immunotherapy side effects is available at NCCN.org/patientguidelines and on the NCCN Patient Guides for Cancer app.

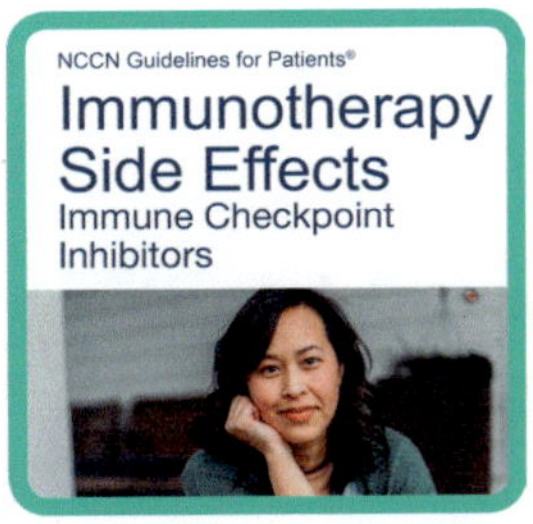

Chemotherapy and systemic therapy are not the same. Systemic therapy includes chemotherapy, targeted therapy, and immunotherapy.

Targeted therapy

Targeted therapy focuses on specific or unique features of cancer cells. Targeted therapies seek out how cancer cells grow, divide, and move in the body. These drugs stop or inhibit the action of molecules that help cancer cells grow and/or survive and are often selected based on NGS and IHC results.

Some examples of targeted therapies include:

- Ramucirumab (Cyramza) targets VEGF (vascular endothelial growth factor) receptors.
- Entrectinib (Rozlytrek) and larotrectinib (Vitrakvi) are examples of TRK inhibitors used for *NTRK* gene fusion-positive tumors.
- Trastuzumab (Herceptin), trastuzumab deruxtecan (Enhertu), or a biosimilar targeting HER2 overexpression-positive tumors.

Radiation therapy

Radiation therapy (RT) uses high-energy radiation from x-rays, photons, protons, electrons, and other sources to kill cancer cells and shrink tumors. RT can be given alone or with other treatments. Unlike how drug therapy travels throughout the whole body to treat a tumor, radiation is a precisely targeted beam on individual areas. It can be targeted on the esophagus containing the tumor, the lymph nodes containing the tumor, as well as nearby areas that may have hidden tumor cells.

RT can be used as the primary treatment for esophageal cancer. It can also be given before or after surgery to treat or slow the growth of cancer, especially if the surgical margins have cancer cells. RT may also be used to treat a tumor that has spread (metastasized) to other parts of your body. RT may also be used as supportive care or palliative care to help ease pain or discomfort caused by cancer, or to control bleeding caused by a tumor.

There are 2 main types of radiation treatment:

- **External beam radiation therapy (EBRT)** uses a machine outside of the body to aim radiation at the tumor(s) or areas of the body.
- **Internal radiation** is placed inside the body as a solid like seeds. This is called brachytherapy.

You won't feel radiation treatments while you're receiving them, but side effects, in the area of the body that is targeted, may develop over time. Discuss the risks and side effects with your care team.

Order of treatments

Most people with cancer will receive more than one type of treatment. Below is an overview of the order of treatments.

- ✓ **Preoperative or neoadjuvant (before) therapy** is given to shrink the tumor before a primary treatment such as surgery.
- ✓ **Perioperative therapy** is systemic therapy, such as chemotherapy, given before and after surgery.
- ✓ **Primary treatment** is the main treatment given to rid the body of cancer.
- ✓ **Postoperative or adjuvant (after) therapy** is given after primary treatment to rid the body of any cancer cells left behind from surgery. It is also used when the risk of cancer returning (recurrence) is felt to be high.
- ✓ **First-line therapy** is the first set of systemic (drug) treatment given.
- ✓ **Second-line therapy** is the next set of treatment given if cancer progresses during or after systemic therapy.

Talk to your care team about your treatment plan and what it means for your stage and type of cancer.

Clinical trials

A clinical trial is a type of medical research study. After being developed and tested in a laboratory, potential new ways of fighting cancer need to be studied in people. If found to be safe and effective in a clinical trial, a drug, device, or treatment approach may be approved by the U.S. Food and Drug Administration (FDA).

Everyone with cancer should carefully consider all of the treatment options available for their cancer type, including standard treatments and clinical trials. Talk to your doctor about whether a clinical trial may make sense for you.

Phases

Most cancer clinical trials focus on treatment. Treatment trials are done in phases.

- **Phase 1** trials study the dose, safety, and side effects of an investigational drug or treatment approach. They also look for early signs that the drug or approach is helpful.
- **Phase 2** trials study how well the drug or approach works against a specific type of cancer.
- **Phase 3** trials test the drug or approach against a standard treatment. If the results are good, it may be approved by the FDA.
- **Phase 4** trials study the long-term safety and benefit of an FDA-approved treatment.

Finding a clinical trial

In the United States

NCCN Cancer Centers
NCCN.org/cancercenters

The National Cancer Institute (NCI)
cancer.gov/about-cancer/treatment/clinical-trials/search

Worldwide

The U.S. National Library of Medicine (NLM)
clinicaltrials.gov

Need help finding a clinical trial?

NCI's Cancer Information Service (CIS)
1.800.4.CANCER (1.800.422.6237)
cancer.gov/contact

Who can enroll?

Every clinical trial has rules for joining, called eligibility criteria. The rules may be about age, cancer type and stage, treatment history, or general health. These requirements ensure that participants are alike in specific ways and that the trial is as safe as possible for the participants.

Informed consent

Clinical trials are managed by a group of experts called a research team. The research team will review the study with you in detail, including its purpose and the risks and benefits of joining. All of this information is also provided in an informed consent form. Read the form carefully and ask questions before signing it. Take time to discuss it with family, friends, or others you trust. Keep in mind that you can leave and seek treatment outside of the clinical trial at any time.

Start the conversation

Don't wait for your doctor to bring up clinical trials. Start the conversation and learn about all of your treatment options. If you find a study that you may be eligible for, ask your treatment team if you meet the requirements. If you have already started standard treatment, you may not be eligible for certain clinical trials. Try not to be discouraged if you cannot join. New clinical trials are always becoming available.

Frequently asked questions

There are many myths and misconceptions surrounding clinical trials. The possible benefits and risks are not well understood by many with cancer.

Will I get a placebo?
Placebos (inactive versions of real medicines) are almost never used alone in cancer clinical trials. It is common to receive either a placebo with a standard treatment or a new drug with a standard treatment. You will be informed, verbally and in writing, if a placebo is part of a clinical trial before you enroll.

Are clinical trials free?
There is no fee to enroll in a clinical trial. The study sponsor pays for research-related costs, including the study drug. You may, however, have costs indirectly related to the trial, such as the cost of transportation or child care due to extra appointments. During the trial, you will continue to receive standard cancer care. This care is billed to—and often covered by—insurance. You are responsible for copays and any costs for this care that are not covered by your insurance.

Supportive care

Supportive care is health care given during all cancer stages. It aims to prevent, reduce, and relieve suffering, and to improve quality of life. Supportive care might include pain relief, emotional or spiritual support, financial aid, or family counseling. Tell your care team how you are feeling and about any side effects so they can be managed. Best supportive care, supportive care, and palliative care are terms that are often used interchangeably.

It is very important to take care of yourself by eating well, drinking plenty of fluids, exercising, and doing activities that make you feel energized. Strength is needed to sustain you during treatment. And as much as you can, you might find it helpful to keep the schedules and activities you had before diagnosis.

After surgery, you may have problems such as getting full too fast, heartburn and reflux, stomach discomfort, bloating, nausea, diarrhea, or dumping syndrome. The feeding tube placed after surgery is usually temporary during the recovery period. Some people also experience discomfort or sticking when swallowing foods. Nutrition plays an important role in managing these symptoms.

Advance care planning

Advance care planning is making decisions now about the care you would want to receive if you become unable to speak for yourself. Advance care planning is for everyone, not just for those who are very sick. It is a way to ensure your wishes are understood and respected.

It is important to tell your care team about all side effects so they can be managed.

Advance care planning starts with an honest discussion with your care team about the course your cancer will take called a prognosis. Find out what you might expect if your cancer spreads or worsens. Discuss the medicines or therapies that will give you the best quality of life and talk about your goals. This dialogue with your care team should be regular (more than once) and will help you achieve your goals in your advance care planning. Include family and friends in your planning, too. Make your wishes clear. It is important that everyone understands what you want.

You don't have to know the exact details of your prognosis. Just having a general idea will help with planning. With this information, you can decide if there is a point where you might want to stop cancer treatment. You can also decide what treatments you would want for symptom relief, such as radiation therapy, surgery, or medicine. You can change your advance care plan at any time. What you want today might change tomorrow. Making your wishes clear will ensure everyone knows what you want.

Bleeding

Bleeding is common in those with esophageal cancer. It may be caused by the tumor or a result of treatment. Endoscopic treatment, radiation therapy (if not done before), or an angiography with embolization might be used to treat (stop) bleeding.

In angiography, a catheter (thin plastic tube) is inserted into an artery through a small incision in the skin and guided to the area with the use of x-rays. A contrast material is injected through the tube and x-ray images produce a picture of the blood vessel called an angiogram. It is often done when a blood vessel has narrowed or suddenly becomes blocked and does not allow blood to flow.

Embolization is the process of blocking blood flow through a blood vessel. This is performed by placing various materials through the angiography catheter while it is inside the blood vessel. The material can be a coil, small beads, or liquid medicine that causes the blood to clot and block the flow of blood.

Blocked esophagus

A tumor may block the esophagus, the esophagogastric junction (EGJ), or the stomach. An esophageal stent is a metal or plastic tube that widens the esophagus so food can pass into the stomach.

Blocked esophagus **An esophageal stent is a tube that widens the esophagus so food can pass into the stomach (image on left). Special expanding (dilating) balloons or bougies can relieve a blockage or a narrowing of the esophagus (image on right).**

Left: https://commons.wikimedia.org/wiki/File:Diagram_showing_an_oesophageal_stent_being_put_in_CRUK_495.svg. Right: https://commons.wikimedia.org/wiki/File:Diagram_showing_how_a_balloon_is_used_to_stretch_the_oesophagus_CRUK_492.svg

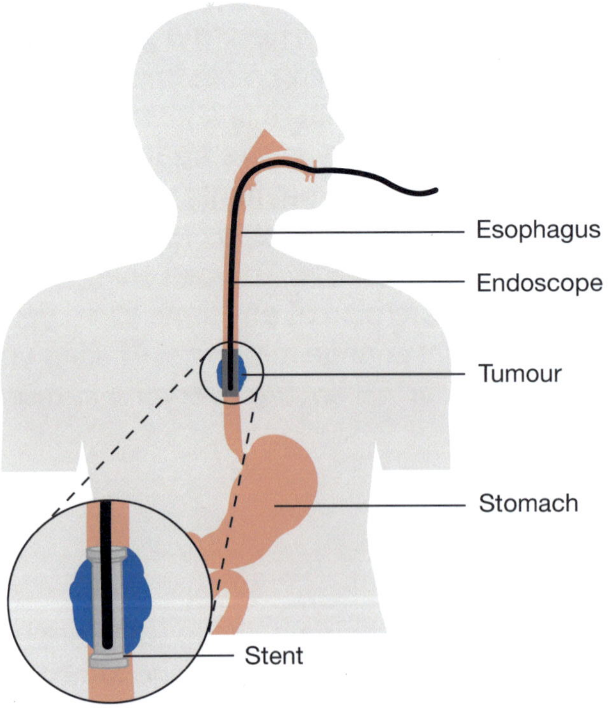

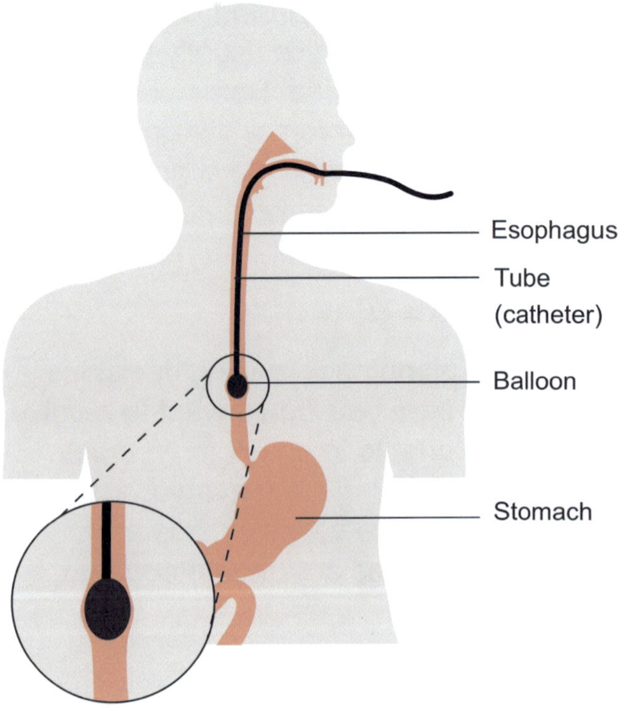

Special expanding (dilating) balloons or bougies can relieve a blockage caused by a tumor or treatment-related narrowing (stricture) of the esophagus. Radiation can also be used to alleviate a blockage.

Difficulty swallowing

Difficult or painful swallowing is called dysphagia. Treatment such as ablation, photodynamic therapy, radiation, or placement of a stent may help relieve pain and discomfort caused by dysphagia.

Eating challenges

Sometimes side effects from surgery, cancer, or other treatments might cause you to feel not hungry or sick to your stomach (nauseated). The tumor may make it difficult to swallow food or liquids. You might have a sore mouth. Healthy eating is important during treatment. It includes eating a balanced diet, eating the right amount of food, and drinking enough fluids. A registered dietitian who is an expert in nutrition and food can help. Medicines are available to treat poor appetite or nausea and vomiting. Speak to your care team if you have trouble eating or maintaining your weight.

For long-term relief of anorexia, dysphagia, or malnutrition, placement of a feeding tube might help.

Supportive care resources

More information on supportive care is available at NCCN.org/patientguidelines and on the NCCN Patient Guides for Cancer app.

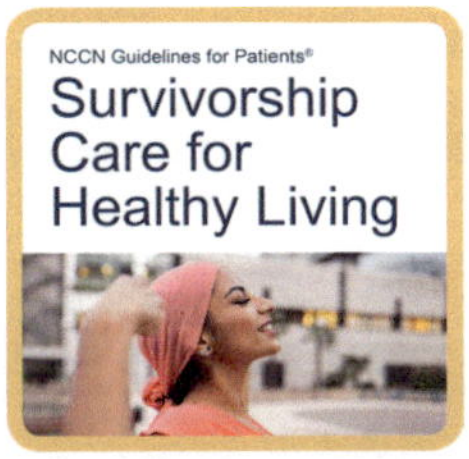

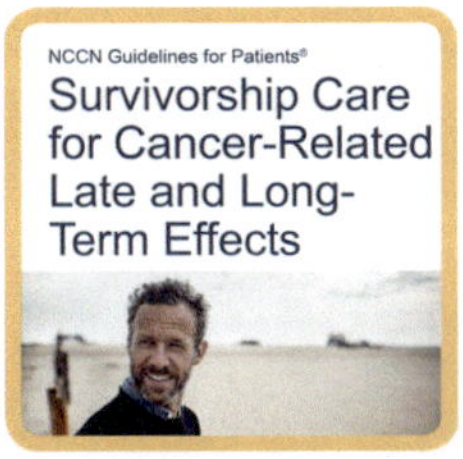

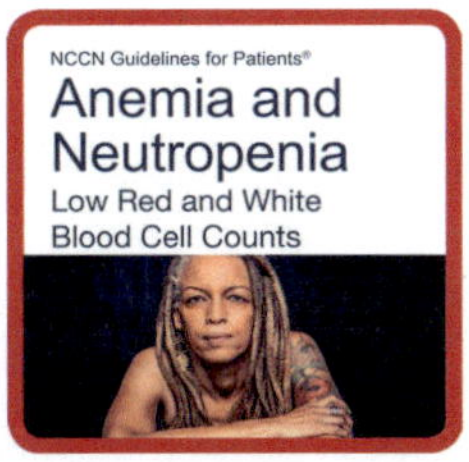

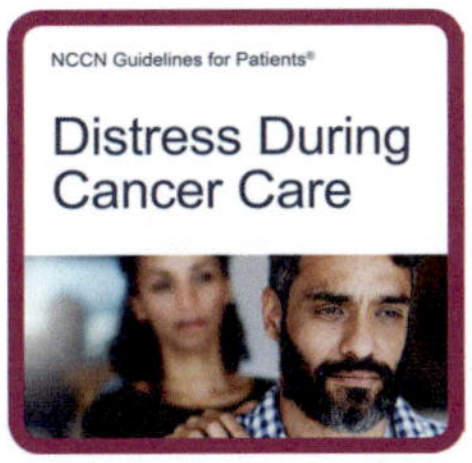

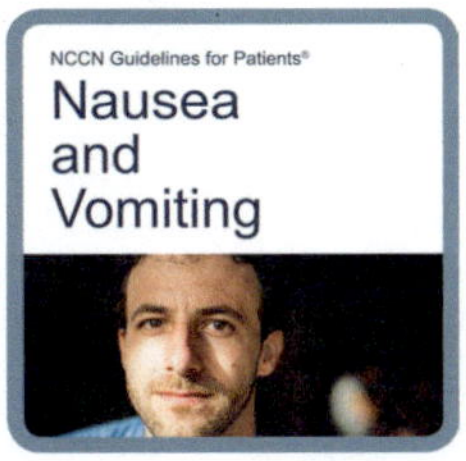

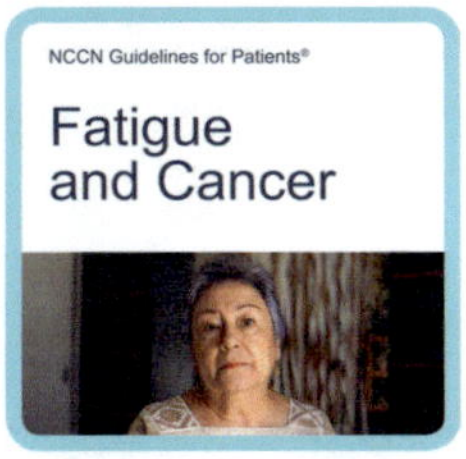

Distress

Distress is an unpleasant experience of a mental, physical, social, or spiritual nature. It can affect how you feel, think, and act. Distress might include feelings of sadness, fear, helplessness, worry, anger, and guilt. Depression, anxiety, and sleeping problems are common in cancer. Talk to your doctor and with those whom you feel most comfortable about how you are feeling. There are services and people who can help you. Support and counseling services are available.

Fatigue

Fatigue is extreme tiredness and inability to function due to lack of energy. Fatigue may be caused by cancer or it may be a side effect of treatment. There are treatments for fatigue. Let your care team know how you are feeling and if fatigue is getting in the way of doing the things you enjoy. Eating a balanced diet, exercise, yoga, acupuncture, and massage therapy can help. You might be referred to a nutritionist or dietitian to help with fatigue.

Nausea and vomiting

Nausea and vomiting are a common side effect of treatment. You will be given medicine to prevent and treat nausea and vomiting.

Pain

Tell your care team about any pain or discomfort. Treating pain can be complicated. You might meet with a palliative care specialist or with a pain specialist to manage pain.

Pain is common in those with a tumor causing a blockage or for metastatic esophageal cancer. Severe abdominal pain can occur when the tumor grows into nearby nerves or presses against other organs. This pain is treated with around-the-clock medicine such as morphine or other opioids (narcotics). Sometimes, non-narcotic medicines are used to treat pain.

Some people may benefit from palliative radiation therapy, with or without systemic therapy, to help relieve the pain. During this treatment, a radiation beam is focused on the tumor.

"My doctor encouraged me to seek additional medical opinions to ensure I was comfortable with my treatment decision. Only after I made up my mind did she share her thoughts."

QOL

Cancer and its treatment can affect your overall well-being or quality of life (QOL). For more information on quality of life, see *NCCN Guidelines for Patients: Palliative Care* at NCCN.org/patientguidelines and on the NCCN Patient Guides for Cancer app.

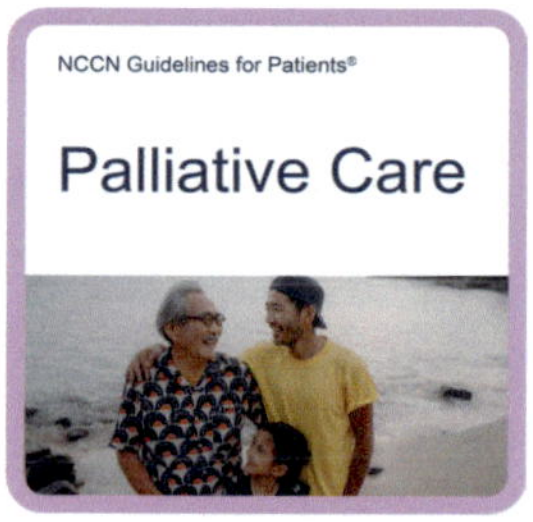

Treatment side effects

All cancer treatments can cause unwanted health issues. Such health issues are called side effects. Side effects depend on many factors. These factors include the drug type and dose, length of treatment, and the person.

Some side effects may be harmful to your health. Others may just be unpleasant.

Ask for a complete list of side effects of your treatments. Also, tell your treatment team about any new or worsening symptoms. There may be ways to help you feel better. There are also ways to prevent some side effects.

Tube feeding

Tube feeding is a special liquid food mixture containing protein, carbohydrates (sugar), fats, vitamins, and minerals, given through a tube. You will likely have tube feeding after surgery to allow your esophagus to heal. The tube is temporary and will be removed. However, some people may need tube feeding for longer periods to maintain weight or for pain or difficulty swallowing.

Liquid nutrition might be given through:

- **A nasogastric tube (NG tube)** inserted through the nose.
- **A gastrostomy tube (G-tube)** placed through the skin of the abdomen directly into the stomach. It is also called a percutaneous endoscopic gastrostomy (PEG) tube.
- **A jejunostomy tube (J-tube)** placed through the skin of the abdomen into the small intestine.

Key points

- Surgery is a main or primary treatment for esophageal cancer.
- A resectable tumor can be removed with surgery. An unresectable tumor cannot be removed with surgery.
- Systemic therapy works throughout the body. It includes chemotherapy, targeted therapy, and immunotherapy.
- Targeted therapies can block the ways cancer cells grow, divide, and move in the body.
- Immunotherapy uses your body's natural defenses to find and destroy cancer cells.
- Radiation therapy (RT) uses high-energy radiation from x-rays, gamma rays, protons, photons, and other sources to kill cancer cells and shrink tumors.
- A clinical trial is a type of research that studies a treatment to see how safe it is and how well it works.

5

Squamous cell carcinoma

Esophageal squamous cell carcinoma (ESCC) starts in the squamous cells of the epithelium, the innermost lining of the esophagus and part of the mucosa. Treatment is based on the size and location of the tumor and your overall health. Together, you and your care team will choose a treatment plan that is best for you.

Esophageal squamous cell carcinoma (ESCC) starts in the thin, flat cells found in the inner lining of the esophagus. Squamous cell carcinoma (SCC) is often found in the upper and middle esophagus. Location is defined by the position of the center of the tumor in the esophagus.

Squamous cell carcinoma location might be described as the cervical (neck region) or non-cervical area of the esophagus. This chapter is for those with early-stage or locoregional (locally advanced) ESCC.

Early stage

Very small early-stage tumors are staged using a biopsy sample from an endoscopic resection. This is called the pathologic stage (pTNM).

Early-stage tumors include:

- pTis – abnormal cells in the epithelium layer of the mucosa
- pT1a – tumor invades lamina propria or muscularis mucosa layer of the mucosa
- pT1b – tumor invades the second layer of the esophagus wall (the submucosa)

Before starting treatment, you might be given liquid nutrition through a tube. Treatment is based on the size, grade, and location of the tumor and your overall health.

Surgery is an option

If you are healthy enough for surgery and do not have any other serious health issues that prevent surgery, then an endoscopic therapy is preferred. An endoscopy therapy might be endoscopic resection (ER) with or without ablation or just ablation. An esophagectomy might be an option as well.

Treatment after a successful endoscopic therapy (tumor completely removed with negative margins) is surveillance. Surveillance consists of testing on a regular basis to watch for signs that cancer has returned. It includes upper GI endoscopy (esophagogastoduodenoscopy or EGD) testing at regular intervals. Other tests might be done.

Treatment after an esophagectomy is based on pathology results and performance status.

Surgery may not be an option

If you are not healthy enough for surgery, the tumor has spread (metastasized), or you do not want surgery, then treatment may include endoscopic resection with or without ablation, or just ablation or chemoradiation.

Treatment after a successful endoscopic therapy (tumor completely removed with negative margins) is surveillance. Surveillance includes upper GI endoscopy (or EGD) testing at regular intervals. Other tests might be done.

Locoregional

In locoregional disease, the tumor has grown into the second layer (submucosa) or other layers of the esophagus. Cancer may be in the lymph nodes. Cancer found in lymph nodes is called node-positive or nodal disease. Lymph nodes must be biopsied or removed to confirm cancer.

Locoregional disease is staged before surgery. This is called clinical stage (cTNM). It is based on endoscopic ultrasound (EUS) and other imaging or biopsy results. Before starting treatment, you might be given liquid nutrition through a tube. Treatment is based on the size, grade, and location of the tumor. Important to note: The cervical esophagus is the upper part of the esophagus or the neck region. The non-cervical esophagus is the mid to lower part of the esophagus.

T = Tumor

A tumor can grow through the layers of the esophagus wall and into nearby structures.

- **Tis tumor** is found in the epithelium (or innermost) layer of the mucosa (first layer).
- **T1a tumor** is found in the lamina propria or muscularis mucosa layers of the mucosa.
- **T1b tumor** is found in the submucosa (second layer).
- **T2 tumor** is found in the muscularis propria (third layer).
- **T3 tumor** is found in the adventitia (outer layer). It has grown through the other layers of the esophagus wall.
- **T4 tumor** has grown all the way through the wall of the esophagus into nearby structures.

Tis and T1 tumors are often considered early-stage cancer. Esophageal cancers are rarely found this early.

T2, T3, and T4 tumors are often referred to as locoregional disease. Cancer may be in lymph nodes or structures near or in direct contact with the esophagus.

In metastatic disease, the tumor can be any size, cancer may be in lymph nodes, and cancer has spread to other parts of the body.

cT1b to T2, N0

An esophagectomy might be an option if the tumor is not in the cervical esophagus, the tumor is less than 3 centimeters (cm), it has not grown beyond the second layer (submucosa) of the esophagus wall, and there is no cancer in the lymph nodes. Treatment after an esophagectomy will be based on the surgical margin results.

cT2 or node-positive tumors

For tumors 3 cm or more, node-positive tumors, or tumors that have grown into or beyond the third layer (muscularis propria) of the esophagus wall, options include:

- Preoperative chemoradiation followed by an esophagectomy
- Chemoradiation alone

After chemoradiation, you will have imaging tests and upper GI endoscopy with biopsy to see if any cancer remains. If no disease remains, then you will enter observation or have an esophagectomy. An esophagectomy is preferred if disease remains.

cT4b

For a tumor that has grown through the layers of the esophagus wall into nearby structures (cT4b), treatment is chemoradiation. Chemotherapy alone might be possible if cancer is found in the trachea (windpipe), large vessels, spine, or heart.

After chemoradiation, you will have imaging tests and upper GI endoscopy with biopsy to see if any cancer remains. An esophagectomy is possible if disease remains or as palliative care. If no disease remains, then you will enter observation.

Standard of care is the best-known way to treat a particular disease based on past clinical trials. There may be more than one treatment regimen that is considered standard of care. Ask your care team what treatment options are available and if a clinical trial might be right for you.

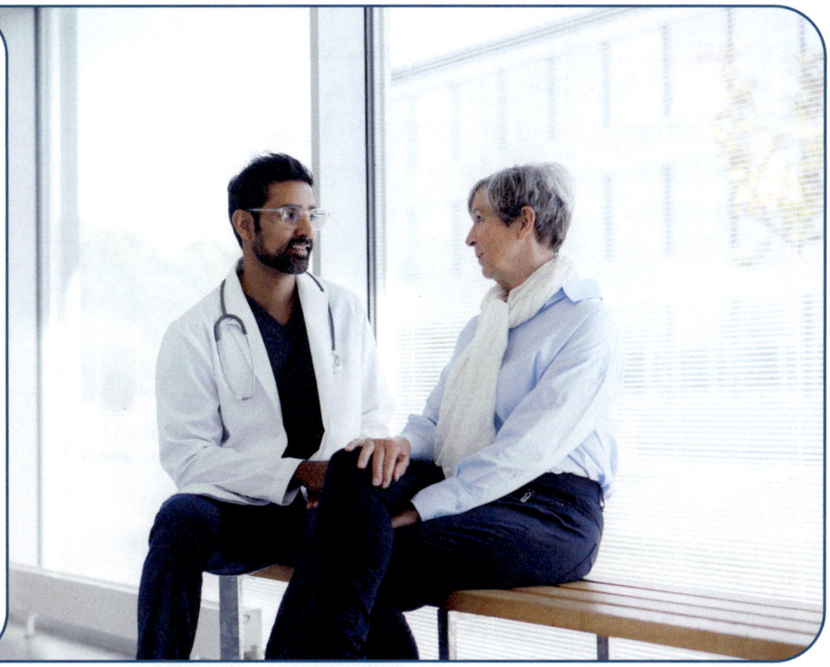

Surgery may not be an option

For those who may not want or are unable to have surgery, chemoradiation, palliative radiation therapy, or palliative care with best supportive care are options. Palliative and best supportive care aim to manage symptoms, improve quality of life, and extend life.

After an esophagectomy

The tumor and lymph nodes removed during surgery will be tested and staged. Treatment after an esophagectomy is also based on if any cancer cells remain in the surgical margin. Options include observation, nivolumab, palliative care, or chemoradiation if you haven't had it before. Palliative care might include systemic therapy and treatment to manage symptoms, improve quality of life, and extend life.

Follow-up care

After treatment, you will receive follow-up care to watch for signs that cancer has returned called recurrence. It is important to keep any follow-up doctor visits and imaging test appointments.

Key points

- Treatment is based on the size and location of the tumor, your overall health, and goals for treatment.
- Very small early-stage tumors have not grown beyond the second layer (submucosa) of the esophagus wall. These are staged using a biopsy sample from an endoscopic resection. This is called the pathologic stage (pTNM).
- Locoregional disease is staged before surgery. This is called clinical stage (cTNM). It is based on endoscopic ultrasound (EUS) and other imaging or biopsy results.
- Your tumor and lymph nodes removed during an esophagectomy will be tested and staged before starting the next treatment.
- Palliative and best supportive care aim to manage symptoms, improve quality of life, and extend life.
- Chemoradiation might be given before (preoperative) or after (postoperative) surgery, or by itself.
- After treatment, you will receive follow-up care. It is important to keep any follow-up doctor visits and imaging test appointments. Contact your doctor if you have any new or worsening symptoms.

6 Adenocarcinoma

Esophageal adenocarcinoma (EAC) starts in the mucus-making cells of the esophagus. Treatment is based on the size and location of the tumor and your overall health. This chapter is for those with early-stage or locoregional (locally advanced) EAC. Together, you and your care team will choose a treatment plan that is best for you.

Early stage

Very small early-stage tumors are staged using a biopsy sample from an endoscopic resection (ER). This is called the pathologic stage (pTNM).

Early-stage tumors include:

- pTis – abnormal cells
- pT1a – tumor invades lamina propria or muscularis mucosa layer of the mucosa
- pT1b – tumor invades submucosa

Before starting treatment, you might be given liquid nutrition through a tube. Treatment is based on the size, grade, and location of the tumor and your overall health.

If you are healthy enough for surgery and do not have any other serious health issues that prevent surgery, then an esophagectomy might be an option. For those who do not want or cannot have surgery, chemoradiation is an option.

Surgery is an option

If you are healthy enough for surgery and do not have any other serious health issues that prevent surgery, then an endoscopic therapy is preferred. An endoscopy therapy might be ER with or without ablation or just ablation. An esophagectomy might be an option as well.

Treatment after an endoscopic therapy is surveillance. Surveillance includes upper GI endoscopy (esophagogastoduodenoscopy or EGD) testing at regular intervals. Other tests might be done.

Surgery may not be an option

A tumor that cannot be completely removed with surgery is called unresectable. For those who have an unresectable tumor, who are medically unable to tolerate major surgery, or who do not want surgery, then treatment will be endoscopic resection and/or ablation. Treatment might be followed by chemoradiation.

Treatment after an endoscopic therapy is surveillance. Surveillance includes upper GI endoscopy (EGD) testing at regular intervals. Other tests might be done.

Locoregional

In locoregional disease, the tumor has grown into the second layer (submucosa) or other layers of the esophagus. Cancer may be in the lymph nodes. Cancer found in lymph nodes is called node-positive or nodal disease. Lymph nodes must be biopsied or removed to confirm cancer.

Locoregional disease is staged before surgery. This is called clinical stage (cTNM). It is based on endoscopic ultrasound (EUS) and other imaging or biopsy results. Before starting treatment, you might be given liquid nutrition through a tube. Treatment is based on the size, grade, and location of the tumor.

cT1b to T2, N0

An esophagectomy might be an option if the tumor is less than 3 centimeters (cm), it has not grown beyond the third layer (muscularis propria) of the esophagus wall, and there is no cancer in the lymph nodes. Treatment after an esophagectomy will be based on the surgical margin results.

cT2 or node-positive tumors

For tumors 3 cm or more, node-positive tumors, or tumors that have grown into or beyond the third layer (muscularis propria) of the esophagus wall, options include:

- Chemoradiation can be done before a planned esophagectomy (preferred). Depending on the results, it might be followed by an esophagectomy.
- Perioperative chemotherapy would be chemotherapy then esophagectomy, followed by chemotherapy.
- If the tumor is MSI-H/dMMR, you might have an immune checkpoint inhibitor (ICI) before (neoadjuvant) and after surgery (perioperatively).
- Chemoradiation is an option for those who do not want an esophagectomy.
- After chemoradiation, you will have imaging tests and upper GI endoscopy with biopsy to see if any cancer remains.

cT4b

For tumor that has grown through the layers of the esophagus wall into nearby structures (cT4b), treatment is chemoradiation. Chemotherapy alone might be possible if cancer is found in the trachea (windpipe), large vessels, spine, or heart.

After treatment, you will have imaging tests and upper GI endoscopy with biopsy to see if any cancer remains. An esophagectomy is possible if disease remains. If no disease remains, then you will enter observation.

Surgery is not an option

Not everyone is healthy enough for or wants surgery. For those who do not want surgery or are not healthy enough for surgery, chemoradiation is an option. Palliative radiation therapy or palliative care with best supportive care are options. Palliative and best supportive care aim to manage symptoms, improve quality of life, and extend life.

Before an esophagectomy

Drug choices before an esophagectomy are based on the type of esophageal cancer, the location of the tumor, and if you might have chemoradiation or systemic therapy after surgery. Ask your care team about the preferred drugs and why one might be chosen over another.

After an esophagectomy

The tumor and lymph nodes removed during surgery will be tested and staged. Treatment options are based on if you had radiation or systemic therapy before surgery and if any cancer remains in the surgical margins.

Options include the following:

- Observation
- Systemic therapy if you received it before surgery
- Chemoradiation if you haven't had radiation therapy before surgery
- Palliative care to manage symptoms, improve quality of life, and extend life

Keep a pain diary

A pain diary is a written record that helps you keep track of when you have pain, how bad it is, what causes it, and what makes it better or worse. Use a pain diary to discuss your pain with your care team. You might be referred to a specialist for pain management.

Include in your pain diary:

- ✓ The time and dose of all medicines
- ✓ When pain starts and ends or lessens
- ✓ Where you feel pain
- ✓ A description of your pain. Is it throbbing, sharp, tingling, shooting, or burning? Is it constant, or does it come and go?
- ✓ Does the pain change at different times of day? When?
- ✓ Does the pain get worse before or after meals? Does certain food or drink make it better?
- ✓ Does the pain get better or worse with activity? What kind of activity?
- ✓ Does the pain keep you from falling asleep at night? Does pain wake you up in the night?
- ✓ A rating of your pain from 0 (no pain) to 10 (worst pain you have ever felt)
- ✓ Does pain get in the way of you doing the things you enjoy?

Follow-up care

After treatment, you will receive follow-up care to watch for signs that cancer has returned. It is important to keep any follow-up doctor visits and imaging test appointments.

> **Cancer can temporarily rob you of your energy, but it can't steal your burning desire to get it all back."**

Key points

- Treatment is based on the size and location of the tumor, your overall health, and goals for treatment.
- Very small early-stage tumors are staged using a biopsy sample from an endoscopic resection. This is called the pathologic stage (pTNM).
- Locoregional disease is staged before surgery. This is called clinical stage (cTNM). It is based on the endoscopic ultrasound (EUS) and other imaging or biopsy results.
- Your tumor and lymph nodes removed during an esophagectomy will be tested and staged before starting the next treatment.
- Chemoradiation might be given before (preoperative) or after (postoperative) surgery, or as definitive treatment.
- Palliative and best supportive care aim to manage symptoms, improve quality of life, and extend life.
- After treatment, you will receive follow-up care. It is important to keep any follow-up doctor visits and imaging test appointments. Contact your doctor if you have any new or worsening symptoms.

7 Recurrent or metastatic disease

This chapter discusses treatment options for recurrent or metastatic disease. Recurrence is the return of cancer. Metastatic cancer is cancer that has spread after being diagnosed or spread after treatment. Together, you and care team will choose a treatment plan that is best for you.

Overview

When cancer returns near the esophagus, it is called locoregional recurrence. Surgery might be an option for those with a locoregional resectable tumor and those who are healthy enough for surgery. Other treatments like palliative care might also be an option.

Esophageal cancer that has spread to distant sites in the body is called metastatic disease. It might be referred to as stage 4 cancer. The most common metastatic sites are the liver, distant lymph nodes, and lung. The goal of treatment is to reduce the amount of cancer, called cancer burden, and to prevent the further spread of cancer.

For unresectable locoregional recurrence, metastatic disease, or those who aren't healthy enough for surgery, treatment will focus on palliative and best supportive care. Systemic therapy might be given. Options are based on biomarker testing status and your performance status (PS). PS is a person's general level of fitness and ability to perform daily tasks.

Your preferences about treatment are always important. Talk to your care team and make your wishes known.

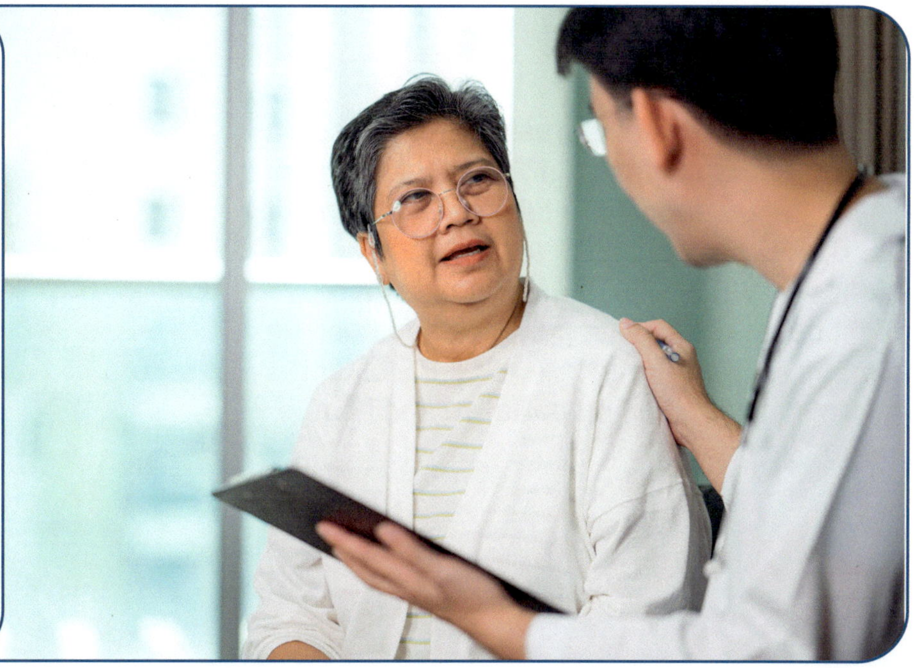

Squamous cell carcinoma

Locoregional recurrence

It is possible to have cancer return in the remaining esophagus. Locoregional recurrence is cancer that has returned to or near the esophagus. Cancer might be in regional lymph nodes.

If you had esophagectomy before, but not chemoradiation

- Treatment options include chemoradiation (preferred), surgery, systemic therapy, or palliative and best supportive care.

If you had chemoradiation before, but not esophagectomy

- If the tumor is resectable and you are healthy enough for surgery, then an esophagectomy is an option.
- If the tumor is unresectable, you are not healthy enough for surgery, or you do not want surgery, then treatment will focus on palliative and best supportive care.

Metastatic disease

For metastatic disease, treatment is based on your performance status (PS) and biomarker testing. If you are able to take care of yourself (PS 0, 1, or 2) and don't have any other serious health issues, then systemic therapy might be an option with palliative and best supportive care. For those with a PS of 3 or 4, treatment focuses on palliative and best supportive care.

Systemic therapy

Systemic therapy might be an option depending on your PS. Before starting systemic therapy, you might have biomarker testing for microsatellite and PD-L1, if not done before and squamous cell carcinoma is suspected.

For systemic therapy options, **see Guide 6** and **Guide 7.**

Guide 6
Squamous cell carcinoma
First-line therapy options: Unresectable, recurrent, or metastatic disease

Preferred options	• Fluoropyrimidine (fluorouracil or capecitabine), oxaliplatin, and nivolumab • Fluoropyrimidine, oxaliplatin, and pembrolizumab • Fluoropyrimidine and oxaliplatin • Fluoropyrimidine, cisplatin, and nivolumab • Fluoropyrimidine, cisplatin, and pembrolizumab • Fluoropyrimidine and cisplatin • Nivolumab and ipilimumab
	MSI-H/dMMR tumors (independent of PD-L1 status) • Pembrolizumab • Dostarlimab-gxly • Nivolumab and ipilimumab • Fluoropyrimidine, oxaliplatin, and nivolumab • Fluoropyrimidine, oxaliplatin, and pembrolizumab
Other recommended	• Fluorouracil and irinotecan • Paclitaxel with or without carboplatin or cisplatin • Docetaxel with or without cisplatin • Fluoropyrimidine • Docetaxel, cisplatin or oxaliplatin, and fluorouracil

Notes: Leucovorin might be added to fluorouracil-based regimens.

Guide 7
Squamous cell carcinoma
Next-line therapy options: Unresectable, recurrent, or metastatic disease

Preferred options	• Nivolumab • Pembrolizumab in some cases • Docetaxel • Paclitaxel • Irinotecan • Tislelizumab-jsgr • Fluorouracil and irinotecan (leucovorin might be added)
Other recommended	• Irinotecan and cisplatin • Docetaxel and irinotecan
Used in some cases	• For *NTRK* gene fusion-positive tumor, entrectinib or larotrectinib • For MSI-H/dMMR tumors, pembrolizumab, nivolumab and ipilimumab, or dostarlimab-gxly • For TMB-H tumors, pembrolizumab • For *BRAF* V600E mutated tumors, dabrafenib or trametinib • For *RET* gene fusion-positive tumors, selpercatinib

Notes: Systemic therapy options are based on prior therapy and performance status (PS).

Adenocarcinoma

Locoregional recurrence

It is possible to have cancer return in the remaining esophagus or to have new cancer in another organ. Locoregional recurrence is cancer that has returned to or near the esophagus. Cancer might be in regional lymph nodes.

If you had esophagectomy before, but not chemoradiation

- Treatment options include chemoradiation (preferred), surgery, systemic therapy, or palliative and best supportive care.

If you had chemoradiation before, but not esophagectomy

- If the tumor is resectable and you are healthy enough for surgery, then an esophagectomy is an option.
- If the tumor is unresectable, you are not healthy enough for surgery, or you do not want surgery, then treatment will focus on palliative and best supportive care.

Metastatic disease

For metastatic disease, treatment is based on your performance status (PS). If you are able to take care of yourself (PS 0, 1, or 2) and don't have any other serious health issues, then systemic therapy might be an option along with palliative and best supportive care. For those with a PS of 3 or 4, treatment focuses on palliative and best supportive care.

A biosimilar or substitute might be used in place of trastuzumab (Herceptin). A biosimilar is an almost identical version of a drug made by another company. It is used in the exact same way and at the same dose as trastuzumab. Biosimilars for trastuzumab include: Kanjinti, Ogivri, Herzuma, Ontruzant, and Trazimera.

Systemic therapy

Systemic therapy might be an option depending on your PS. Before starting systemic therapy, you might have biomarker testing for microsatellite, PD-L1, and HER2 tumor testing if not done before and adenocarcinoma is suspected.

For systemic therapy options, **see Guide 8** and **Guide 9.**

Guide 8
Adenocarcinoma
First-line therapy options: Unresectable, recurrent, or metastatic disease

Preferred options	For HER2 overexpression-positive tumors: • Fluoropyrimidine (fluorouracil or capecitabine), oxaliplatin, and trastuzumab • Fluoropyrimidine and oxaliplatin, trastuzumab, and pembrolizumab • Fluoropyrimidine, cisplatin, and trastuzumab • Fluoropyrimidine, cisplatin, trastuzumab, and pembrolizumab
	For HER2 overexpression-negative tumors: • Fluoropyrimidine, oxaliplatin, and nivolumab • Fluoropyrimidine, oxaliplatin, and pembrolizumab • Fluoropyrimidine and oxaliplatin • Fluoropyrimidine, cisplatin, and pembrolizumab • Fluoropyrimidine and cisplatin
	MSI-H/dMMR tumors (independent of PD-L1 status): • Pembrolizumab • Dostarlimab-gxly • Nivolumab and ipilimumab • Fluoropyrimidine, oxaliplatin, and nivolumab • Fluoropyrimidine, oxaliplatin, and pembrolizumab
Other recommended	• Fluorouracil and irinotecan • Paclitaxel with or without carboplatin or cisplatin • Docetaxel with or without cisplatin • Fluoropyrimidine (fluorouracil or capecitabine) • Docetaxel, cisplatin or oxaliplatin, and fluorouracil

Notes: An FDA-approved biosimilar might be used for trastuzumab. Leucovorin might be added to fluorouracil-based regimens.

Guide 9
Adenocarcinoma
Next-line therapy options: Unresectable, recurrent, or metastatic disease

Preferred options	• Ramucirumab and paclitaxel • Fam-trastuzumab deruxtecan-nxki for HER2 overexpression positive • Docetaxel • Paclitaxel • Irinotecan • Fluorouracil and irinotecan • Trifluridine and tipiracil for third-line or subsequent therapy for esophagogastric junction (EGJ) adenocarcinoma
Other recommended	• Ramucirumab • Irinotecan and cisplatin • Fluorouracil and irinotecan with ramucirumab (leucovorin might be added) • Irinotecan and ramucirumab • Docetaxel and irinotecan
Used in some cases	• Entrectinib or larotrectinib for *NTRK* gene fusion-positive tumor • For MSI-H/dMMR tumors, pembrolizumab, nivolumab and ipilimumab, or dostarlimab-gxly • Pembrolizumab for TMB-H tumors • Dabrafenib and trametinib for *BRAF* V600E mutated tumors • Selpercatinib for *RET* gene fusion-positive tumors

Notes: Systemic therapy options are based on prior therapy and performance status (PS).

Key points

- It is possible to have cancer return in the remaining esophagus or to have recurrent cancer in another organ (metastasis).
- Locoregional recurrence is cancer that has returned to or near the esophagus. Cancer might be in regional lymph nodes.
- Esophageal cancer that has spread to distant sites in the body is called metastatic disease. It might be referred to as stage 4 cancer.
- The most common metastatic sites are the liver, distant lymph nodes, and lung.
- The goal of treatment is to reduce the amount of cancer, called cancer burden, and to prevent the further spread of cancer.
- An unresectable tumor cannot be completely removed with surgery.
- Treatment for an unresectable and/or metastatic disease is palliative and best supportive care with or without systemic therapy, depending on your performance status (PS).

share with us.

Take our survey and help make the NCCN Guidelines for Patients better for everyone!

NCCN.org/patients/comments

8

Survivorship

After treatment, you will be monitored for any new or ongoing health issues. It is important to keep any follow-up doctor visits and imaging test appointments. Maintain your weight, eat a healthy diet, exercise, limit alcohol, and if you smoke or vape, seek help to quit.

Monitoring

In addition to monitoring for the possible return of cancer called recurrence, you should seek good routine medical care, including regular doctor visits for preventive care and cancer screening. Routine esophageal cancer-specific tests such as imaging, endoscopy, or tumor tests are not recommended after 5 years. It is important to keep any follow-up doctor visits and imaging test appointments.

General health

Esophageal cancer survivors are monitored for long-term side effects. Side effects can be managed. Talk to your doctor about how you are feeling.

In general:

- Maintain a healthy body weight throughout life.
- Adopt a physically active lifestyle. The goal is at least 30 minutes of moderate-intensity activity most days of the week.
- Eat a mostly plant-based diet.
- Limit alcohol.
- If you smoke or vape, seek help to quit.

You might find it helpful to talk to your care team about survivorship resources in your area. For more information on survivorship, see *NCCN Guidelines for Patients: Survivorship Care* at NCCN.org/patientguidelines and on the NCCN Patient Guides for Cancer app.

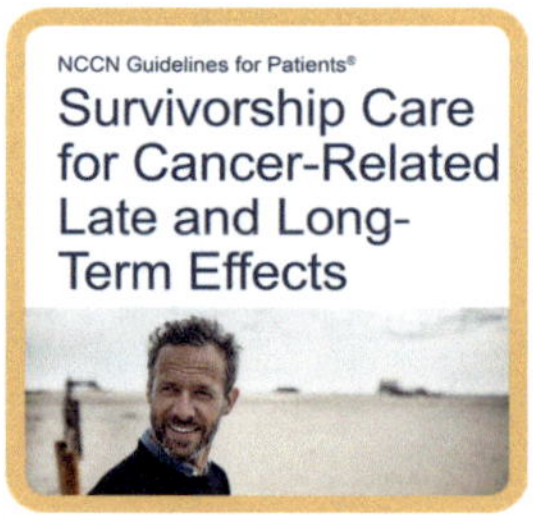

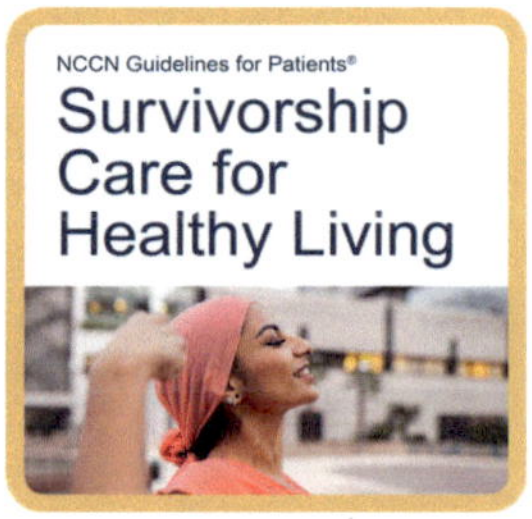

Diarrhea

Diarrhea is frequent and watery bowel movements. Your care team will tell you how to manage diarrhea and may recommend medicines to stop the diarrhea. It is important to drink lots of fluids. Changes to your diet might help.

Difficulty swallowing

Dysphagia or difficulty swallowing may be a result of an esophagectomy. When part of the esophagus is surgically removed, the two remaining ends are sewn or stapled together (anastomosed). An anastomotic stricture (or stenosis) is a narrowing of the esophagus after an esophagectomy. This can be managed with endoscopic dilation.

Dumping syndrome

Dumping syndrome occurs when food empties into the small intestine too quickly. This may happen within 30 minutes after eating a meal (early dumping syndrome) or within 2 to 3 hours of eating (late dumping syndrome).

Symptoms of early dumping syndrome include palpitations, diarrhea, nausea, and cramps. Late dumping syndrome tends to cause dizziness, hunger, cold sweats, and faintness.

To help manage the symptoms of dumping syndrome:

- Eat often throughout the day.
- Avoid drinking liquids with meals.
- Eat a diet high in protein and fiber and low in simple carbohydrates and sugars.

Fatigue

Fatigue is extreme tiredness and inability to function due to lack of energy. There are treatments for fatigue. Let your care team know how you are feeling and if fatigue is getting in the way of doing the things you enjoy. A balanced diet, exercise, yoga, and massage therapy can help. You might be referred to a nutritionist or dietitian to help with fatigue.

Fullness after meals and eating issues

Eat small portions and eat more often to cope with feeling full after meals. Minimize high fat and high fiber content in food. Also, avoid drinking liquids with meals. Continue to drink fluids in between meals. You might be referred to a gastroenterologist for ongoing symptoms.

Heart issues

Because of the location of the esophagus, radiation therapy for esophageal cancer may cause heart issues. You should work with your primary care doctor to monitor your blood pressure, cholesterol, blood sugar, and weight.

Indigestion

Indigestion is a general term that describes discomfort in your upper abdomen. Indigestion is also called dyspepsia or an upset stomach.

To prevent indigestion, avoid foods that increase acid production such as citrus juices, tomato sauces, and spicy foods.

Neuropathy

Neuropathy is a nerve problem that causes pain, numbness, tingling, swelling, or muscle weakness in different parts of the body. It usually begins in the hands or feet and gets worse over time. Neuropathy caused by chemotherapy is called chemotherapy-induced neuropathy.

Reflux

Reflux is the backward flow of liquid from the stomach into the esophagus. Avoid lying flat after eating. Use a foam wedge (triangular) pillow in bed and sleep in a slightly upright position at night. Talk to your doctor before taking any over-the-counter (OTC) medicine. Do not eat within 2 hours of bedtime.

Weight loss

Your weight will be monitored for changes. You might weigh less after an esophagectomy. Weight loss is expected in the first 6 months after surgery. In addition, you will be monitored to make sure you are getting enough nutrition, and your body is absorbing the nutrition from the food you eat.

Healthy eating is very important. It includes eating a balanced diet, eating the right amount of food, and drinking enough fluids. Eat often and avoid fluids with meals.

A registered dietitian who is an expert in nutrition and food can help if you have trouble eating, absorbing nutrition, or maintaining weight.

Cancer screening

Schedule cancer screenings and vaccinations as recommended by your doctor based on your age, risk, and other factors.

Screenings for cancer include:

- Breast
- Colorectal
- Lung
- Prostate

Key points

- Surgery and other treatments for esophageal cancer can cause health issues. Your health will be monitored.
- A nutritionist or dietician provides guidance on what foods are most suitable for your condition.
- Continue to see your primary health care provider on a regular basis and have preventive cancer screenings as recommended by your doctor.
- Eat often throughout the day (graze) and avoid drinking liquids with meals.
- Eat a mostly plant-based diet that is high in protein and fiber and low in simple carbohydrates and sugars.
- Limit alcohol.
- If you smoke or vape, seek help to quit.

9

Making treatment decisions

It's important to be comfortable with the cancer treatment you choose. This choice starts with having an open and honest conversation with your care team.

It's your choice

In shared decision-making, you and your care team share information, discuss the options, and agree on a treatment plan. It starts with an open and honest conversation between you and your care team.

Treatment decisions are very personal. What is important to you may not be important to someone else. Some things that may play a role in your decision-making:

- What you want and how that might differ from what others want
- Your religious and spiritual beliefs
- Your feelings about certain treatments
- Your feelings about pain or side effects
- Cost of treatment, travel to treatment centers, and time away from school or work
- Quality of life and length of life
- How active you are and the activities that are important to you

Think about what you want from treatment. Discuss openly the risks and benefits of specific treatments and procedures. Weigh options and share concerns with your care team. If you take the time to build a relationship with your care team, it will help you feel supported when considering options and making treatment decisions.

Second opinion

It is normal to want to start treatment as soon as possible. While cancer can't be ignored, there is time to have another doctor review your test results and suggest a treatment plan. This is called getting a second opinion, and it's a normal part of cancer care. Even doctors get second opinions!

Things you can do to prepare:

- Check with your insurance company about its rules on second opinions. There may be out-of-pocket costs to see doctors who are not part of your insurance plan.
- Make plans to have copies of all your records sent to the doctor you will see for your second opinion.

Support groups

Many people diagnosed with cancer find support groups to be helpful. Support groups often include people at different stages of treatment. Some people may be newly diagnosed, while others may be finished with treatment. If your hospital or community doesn't have support groups for people with cancer, check out the websites listed in this book.

Questions to ask

Possible questions to ask your care team are listed on the following pages. Feel free to use these questions or come up with your own.

Questions about cancer testing

1. What tests will I have?
2. Do the tests have any risks?
3. Will my insurance pay for this test?
4. Do I need to do anything to prepare for testing?
5. Should I bring someone with me to the appointments?
6. Where do I go for testing, and how long will it take?
7. If any of the tests will hurt, what will you do to make me comfortable?
8. How soon will I know the results and who will explain them to me?
9. How can I get a copy of the pathology report and other test results?
10. Is there an online portal with my test results?

Questions about your care team's experience

1. What is your experience treating esophageal cancer? What else do you treat?
2. What is the experience of those on your team?
3. Does your center discuss cases in a multidiscipliary tumor board conference?
4. How many people with my same stage and type of cancer have you treated? What is the rate of survival?
5. Will you be consulting with experts to discuss my care? Whom will you consult?
6. How many esophageal procedures like the one you're suggesting have you done?
7. How many of your patients have had complications? What were the complications?
8. How much time can I expect to spend with my care team in outpatient visits?
9. Who will manage my day-to-day care?
10. I would like a second opinion. Is there someone you can recommend?

Questions about treatment options

1. What are my treatment options?
2. What is the stage of my disease?
3. Is a clinical trial an option for me?
4. What will happen if I do nothing?
5. How do my age, sex, overall health, and other factors affect my options?
6. What if I am pregnant, or planning to become pregnant?
7. Does any option offer a cure or long-term cancer control?
8. What are the side effects of the treatments?
9. I would like a second opinion. Is there someone you can recommend?
10. How long do I have to decide about treatment, and is there a social worker or someone else who can help me decide?

Questions about what to expect

1. Why do you think this hospital or cancer center offers the best treatment for me?
2. Do I have a choice of when to begin treatment?
3. How long will treatment last?
4. Will my insurance cover the treatment you're recommending?
5. Are there any programs to help pay for treatment?
6. What supportive care and services are available to me and my caregivers?
7. Who should I contact with questions or concerns if the office is closed?
8. How will you know if treatment is working?
9. What are the chances of the cancer worsening or returning?
10. What follow-up care is needed after treatment?

Questions about side effects

1. What are the possible complications and side effects of treatment?
2. Does the cancer itself cause any side effects?
3. Which side effects are most common and how long do they usually last?
4. Which side effects are serious or life-threatening?
5. Are there any long-term or permanent side effects?
6. What symptoms should I report right away, and who do I contact?
7. What can I do to prevent or relieve the side effects of treatment?
8. Do any medications worsen side effects?
9. How will my quality of life be affected by treatment? What are the tradeoffs?
10. Will you stop or change treatment if there are serious side effects?

Questions about clinical trials

1. Do you recommend that I consider a clinical trial for treatment?
2. How do I find clinical trials that I can participate in?
3. What are the treatments used in the clinical trial?
4. Has the treatment been used for other types of cancer?
5. What are the risks and benefits of this treatment?
6. What side effects should I expect and how will they be managed?
7. How long will I be in the clinical trial?
8. Will I be able to get other treatment if this doesn't work?
9. How will you know if the treatment is working?
10. Will the clinical trial cost me anything?

Questions about resources and support

1. Who can I talk to about help with housing, food, and other basic needs?
2. What assistance is available for transportation, childcare, and home care?
3. How much will I have to pay for treatment?
4. What help is available to pay for medicines and other treatment?
5. What other services are available to me and my caregivers?
6. How can I connect with others and build a support system?
7. How can I find in-person or online support?
8. Who can help me with my concerns about missing work or school?
9. Who can I talk to if I don't feel safe at home, at work, or in my neighborhood?
10. How can I get help to stop smoking or vaping?

Resources

Bone Marrow & Cancer Foundation
Bonemarrow.org

Cancer*Care*
Cancercare.org

Cancer Hope Network
Cancerhopenetwork.org

ECAN Esophageal Cancer Action Network
ecan.org

Esophageal Cancer Awareness Association dba EC Aware
ecaware.org

Esophageal Cancer Education Foundation
fightec.org

Imerman Angels
Imermanangels.org

MedlinePlus
medlineplus.gov/esophagealcancer.html

National Cancer Institute
cancer.gov/types/esophageal

National Coalition for Cancer Survivorship
canceradvocacy.org

Triage Cancer
Triagecancer.org

Words to know

abdomen
The belly area between the chest and pelvis.

adenocarcinoma
Cancer cells that form glands and may produce mucus.

anastomotic stricture (or stenosis)
Narrowing of the esophagus after an esophagectomy.

Barrett esophagus (BE)
A condition in which the cells lining the lower part of the esophagus have changed or been replaced with abnormal cells that could lead to cancer of the esophagus.

best supportive care
Treatment that improves quality of life.

biopsy
A procedure that removes fluid or tissue samples to be tested for a disease.

biosimilar
A drug that is very much like one that has been approved by the U.S. Food and Drug Administration (FDA). It must be used in the exact same way and at the same dose as the other drug.

brachytherapy
A treatment with radiation from an object placed near or in the tumor. Also called internal radiation.

bronchi
The two airways extending from the windpipe into the lungs.

bronchoscope
A device that is guided through the nose or mouth to examine the inside of the trachea, bronchi, and lungs.

cancer grade
A rating of how much cancer cells look like normal cells.

cancer stage
A rating of the growth and spread of cancer.

cardia
The part of the stomach that is closest to the esophagus. Food and liquids pass through the cardia to enter the stomach from the esophagus.

carina
A ridge at the base of the trachea (windpipe) that separates the openings of the right and left main bronchi (the large air passages that lead from the trachea to the lungs).

chemoradiation
Treatment that combines chemotherapy with radiation therapy.

chemotherapy
Drugs that kill cancer cells by damaging or disrupting the making of the genetic code.

clinical stage (c)
Rating the extent of a tumor based on tests before treatment.

clinical trial
Research on a test or treatment to assess its safety or how well it works.

colon
The longest part of the large intestine.

complete blood count (CBC)
A test of the number of blood cells.

comprehensive chemistry profile
A panel of tests that gives information about the health and functions of the kidneys and the liver. Usually ordered as part of a comprehensive metabolic panel (CMP).

computed tomography (CT)
A test that uses x-rays to view body parts.

conduit
Tube-shaped tissue, such as the stomach or part of the colon or small intestine, that replaces the part of the esophagus removed during an esophagectomy.

contrast
A substance put into your body to make clearer pictures during imaging tests.

definitive treatment
The best treatment after all choices have been considered.

diaphragm
The thin muscle below the lungs and heart that separates the chest from the abdomen and helps a person to breathe.

digestive system
A set of organs that breaks down food for the body to use.

digestive tract
A set of tube-shaped organs that breaks down food for the body to use. Part of the digestive system.

duodenum
First part of the small intestine.

dysphagia
Difficult or painful swallowing.

Eastern Cooperative Oncology Group (ECOG) Performance Scale
A rating scale of one's ability to do daily activities.

endoscope
A thin, long tube fitted with tools that is guided down the mouth.

endoscopic mucosal resection (EMR)
Removal of early tumors with a snare that has been guided down the throat.

endoscopic resection (ER)
Treatment that removes early tumors with a tool guided down the throat.

endoscopic submucosal dissection (ESD)
Removal of early tumors with a special knife that has been guided down the throat.

endoscopic ultrasound (EUS)
A device guided down your throat to make pictures using sound waves.

epithelium
Cells that line the esophagus wall.

esophagectomy
A surgery that removes all or part of the esophagus.

esophagogastroduodenoscopy (EGD)
Use of a thin tool guided down the throat into the esophagus and stomach. Also called an upper endoscopy or upper gastrointestinal (GI) endoscopy.

esophagogastrostomy
A surgery that removes the esophagus and some of the stomach.

esophagogastric junction (EGJ)
The area where the esophagus and stomach join.

esophagus
The tube-shaped organ between the throat and stomach.

external beam radiation therapy (EBRT)
Radiation therapy received from a machine outside the body.

fine-needle aspiration (FNA)
Removal of a tissue sample with a thin needle.

gastroenterologist
A doctor who's an expert in digestive diseases.

gastrointestinal (GI) tract
The group of organs through which food passes after being eaten. Also called digestive tract.

gastrostomy tube (G-tube)
A feeding tube that is inserted through a cut in the skin of the abdomen directly into the stomach. Also called a percutaneous endoscopic gastrostomy (PEG) tube.

general anesthesia
A loss of feeling and a complete loss of awareness that feels like a very deep sleep.

hereditary
Passed down from birth parent to child through coded information in cells.

high-grade dysplasia (HGD)
Abnormal cells that are likely to become cancer cells.

human epidermal growth factor receptor 2 (HER2)
A protein on the surface of a cell that sends signals for the cell to grow.

jejunostomy tube (J-tube)
A feeding tube that is inserted through a cut into the middle intestine (jejunum).

jejunum
The middle part of the small intestine.

imaging
A test that makes pictures (images) of the insides of the body.

immune system
The body's natural defense against infection and disease.

immunotherapy
A treatment with drugs that help the body find and destroy cancer cells.

infection
An illness caused by germs.

interventional radiologist
A doctor who is an expert in imaging tests and using image-guided tools to perform minimally invasive techniques to diagnose or treat disease.

intestine
The organ that food passes through after leaving the stomach.

intravenous (IV)
A method of giving drugs by a needle or tube inserted into a vein.

Karnofsky Performance Status (KPS)
A rating scale of one's ability to do daily activities.

lamina propria
Connective tissue within the mucosa of the esophagus wall.

laparoscopy
Use of a thin tool inserted through a cut made into the belly area.

lymph
A clear fluid containing white blood cells.

lymph node
A small group of special disease-fighting cells located throughout the body.

lymph node dissection
A type of surgery that removes some disease-fighting structures called lymph nodes.

medical oncologist
A doctor who's an expert in cancer drugs.

metastasis
The spread of cancer cells from the first (primary) tumor to a new site.

microsatellite instability (MSI)
Errors made in small, repeated DNA parts during the copy process because of an abnormal repair system.

microsatellite instability-high (MSI-H)
Mutations in 30% or more microsatellites.

minimally invasive procedure
A procedure that uses small incisions or a tool placed into the opening of the body to reduce damage to body tissue.

mucosa
The first, inner layer of the esophagus wall. It is made up of 3 layers: epithelium, lamina propria, and muscularis mucosa.

muscularis mucosa
A thin layer of muscle separating the mucosa from the submucosa of the esophagus wall.

muscularis propria
The third layer of the esophagus wall made mostly of muscle.

mutation
An abnormal change.

nasogastric tube (NG tube)
Inserted through the nose and into the stomach to provide liquid nutrition.

observation
A period of testing for changes in cancer status while not receiving treatment.

palliative care
Care given to improve the quality of life and help reduce suffering.

pathologic stage (p)
A rating of the extent of cancer based on microscopic review after treatment.

pathologist
A doctor who's an expert in examining tissue and cells to find disease.

pelvis
The area of the body between the hip bones.

percutaneous endoscopic gastrostomy (PEG)
A procedure that inserts a feeding tube into the stomach through a small cut in the skin.

positron emission tomography-computed tomography (PET/CT)
A test that uses radioactive material and x-rays to see the shape and function of body parts.

primary treatment
The main treatment used to rid the body of cancer.

primary tumor
The first mass of cancer cells.

radiation oncologist
A doctor who's an expert in radiation treatment.

radiation therapy (RT)
A treatment that uses high-energy rays.

radiologist
A doctor who is an expert in imaging tests.

recurrence
The return of cancer after a cancer-free period.

resectable
Cancer that can be removed with surgery.

side effect
An unhealthy or unpleasant physical or emotional response to treatment.

small intestine
The digestive organ that absorbs nutrients from eaten food.

squamous cell carcinoma (SCC)
A type of cancer that starts in thin and flat cells that line the surface of organs like the esophagus.

stricture
Narrowing of the esophagus. Might be caused by a tumor or treatment.

submucosa
The second layer of the esophagus wall made mostly of connective tissue, blood vessels, and nerve cells.

subtype
A smaller group within a type of cancer that is based on certain cell features.

supportive care
Health care that includes symptom relief but not cancer treatment. Also called palliative care.

surgical margin
The normal-looking tissue around the edge of a tumor that is removed during surgery.

surgical oncologist
A surgeon who's an expert in performing surgical procedures in people with cancer.

surveillance
Testing after treatment ends to check for the return of cancer.

targeted therapy
Drugs that stop the growth process specific to cancer cells.

trachea
The airway between the throat and airway into the lungs. Also called the windpipe.

tumor marker
A substance found in body tissue or fluid that may be a sign of cancer.

tunica adventitia
The outermost layer of the esophagus wall.

ultrasound (US)
A test that uses sound waves to take pictures of the insides of the body.

unresectable
Cancer that can't be removed by surgery.

upper endoscopy
Use of a thin tool guided down the throat into the esophagus and stomach. Also called an upper gastrointestinal (GI) endoscopy or esophagogastroduodenoscopy (EGD).

widespread metastatic disease
The spread of cancer from the first tumor to many new sites in the body.

NCCN Contributors

This patient guide is based on the NCCN Clinical Practice Guidelines in Oncology (NCCN Guidelines®) for Esophageal and Esophagogastric Junction Cancers, Version 2.2024. It was adapted, reviewed, and published with help from the following people:

Dorothy A. Shead, MS
Senior Director
Patient Information Operations

Tanya Fischer
Senior Medical Writer

Christine McLaughlin
Medical Writer

Laura Phillips
Graphic Artist

The NCCN Clinical Practice Guidelines in Oncology (NCCN Guidelines®) for Esophageal and Esophagogastric Junction Cancers, Version 2.2024 were developed by the following NCCN Panel Members:

*Jaffer A. Ajani, MD/Chair
The University of Texas
MD Anderson Cancer Center

*Thomas A. D'Amico, MD/Vice Chair
Duke Cancer Institute

*Afsaneh Barzi, MD, PhD
City of Hope National Medical Center

David J. Bentrem, MD, MS
Robert H. Lurie Comprehensive Cancer Center of Northwestern University

David T. Cooke, MD
UC Davis Comprehensive Cancer Center

Carlos Corvera, MD
UCSF Helen Diller Family Comprehensive Cancer Center

Prajnan Das, MD, MS, MPH
The University of Texas
MD Anderson Cancer Center

Peter C. Enzinger, MD
Dana-Farber/Brigham and Women's Cancer Center

Thomas Enzler, MD, PhD
University of Michigan Rogel Cancer Center

Hans Gerdes, MD
Memorial Sloan Kettering Cancer Center

*Michael K. Gibson, MD, PhD
Vanderbilt-Ingram Cancer Center

Patrick Grierson, MD, PhD
Siteman Cancer Center at Barnes-Jewish Hospital and Washington University School of Medicine

Wayne L. Hofstetter, MD
The University of Texas
MD Anderson Cancer Center

David H. Ilson, MD, PhD
Memorial Sloan Kettering Cancer Center

Shadia Jalal, MD
Indiana University Melvin and Bren Simon Comprehensive Cancer Center

Rajesh Keswani, MD
Robert H. Lurie Comprehensive Cancer Center of Northwestern University

*Sunnie Kim, MD
University of Colorado Cancer Center

*Lawrence R. Kleinberg, MD
The Sidney Kimmel Comprehensive Cancer Center at Johns Hopkins

*Samuel Klempner, MD
Mass General Cancer Center

Jill Lacy, MD
Yale Cancer Center/Smilow Cancer Hospital

Byrne Lee, MD
Stanford Cancer Institute

*Frank Licciardi, patient advocate
Memorial Sloan Kettering Cancer Center

Shane Lloyd, MD
Huntsman Cancer Institute at the University of Utah

Quan P. Ly, MD
Fred & Pamela Buffett Cancer Center

Kristina A. Matkowskyj, MD, PhD
University of Wisconsin Carbone Cancer Center

Michael McNamara, MD
Case Comprehensive Cancer Center/ University Hospitals Seidman Cancer Center and Cleveland Clinic Taussig Cancer Institute

Ryan Merkow, MD, MS
The UChicago Medicine Comprehensive Cancer Center

Aaron Miller, MD, PhD
UC San Diego Moores Cancer Center

Sarbajit Mukherjee, MD, MS
Roswell Park Comprehensive Cancer Center

Mary F. Mulcahy, MD
Robert H. Lurie Comprehensive Cancer Center of Northwestern University

Darryl Outlaw, MD
O'Neal Comprehensive Cancer Center at UAB

Kyle A. Perry, MD
The Ohio State University Comprehensive Cancer Center - James Cancer Hospital and Solove Research Institute

*Jose Pimiento, MD
Moffitt Cancer Center

George A. Poultsides, MD, MS
Stanford Cancer Institute

Deepti Reddi, MD
Fred Hutchinson Cancer Center

*Scott Reznik, MD
UT Southwestern Simmons Comprehensive Cancer Center

Robert E. Roses, MD
Abramson Cancer Center at the University of Pennsylvania

Vivian E. Strong, MD
Memorial Sloan Kettering Cancer Center

Stacy Su, MD
Fox Chase Cancer Center

Nataliya Uboha, MD, PhD
University of Wisconsin Carbone Cancer Center

Zev Wainberg, MD
UCLA Jonsson Comprehensive Cancer Center

Hanlin L. Wang, MD, PhD
UCLA Jonsson Comprehensive Cancer Center

Georgia Wiesner, MD/Liaison
Vanderbilt-Ingram Cancer Center

Christopher G. Willett, MD
Duke Cancer Institute

Harry Yoon, MD
Mayo Clinic Comprehensive Cancer Center

NCCN

Lisa Hang, PhD
Oncology Scientist/Senior Medical Writer

Nicole McMillian, MS
Senior Guidelines Coordinator

MaryElizabeth Stein, PhD
Associate Scientist/Medical Writer

* Reviewed this patient guide. For disclosures, visit NCCN.org/disclosures.

NCCN Cancer Centers

Abramson Cancer Center
at the University of Pennsylvania
Philadelphia, Pennsylvania
800.789.7366 • pennmedicine.org/cancer

Case Comprehensive Cancer Center/
University Hospitals Seidman Cancer Center and
Cleveland Clinic Taussig Cancer Institute
Cleveland, Ohio
UH Seidman Cancer Center
800.641.2422 • uhhospitals.org/services/cancer-services
CC Taussig Cancer Institute
866.223.8100 • my.clevelandclinic.org/departments/cancer
Case CCC
216.844.8797 • case.edu/cancer

City of Hope National Medical Center
Duarte, California
800.826.4673 • cityofhope.org

Dana-Farber/Brigham and Women's Cancer Center |
Mass General Cancer Center
Boston, Massachusetts
877.442.3324 • youhaveus.org
617.726.5130 • massgeneral.org/cancer-center

Duke Cancer Institute
Durham, North Carolina
888.275.3853 • dukecancerinstitute.org

Fox Chase Cancer Center
Philadelphia, Pennsylvania
888.369.2427 • foxchase.org

Fred & Pamela Buffett Cancer Center
Omaha, Nebraska
402.559.5600 • unmc.edu/cancercenter

Fred Hutchinson Cancer Center
Seattle, Washington
206.667.5000 • fredhutch.org

Huntsman Cancer Institute at the University of Utah
Salt Lake City, Utah
800.824.2073 • healthcare.utah.edu/huntsmancancerinstitute

Indiana University Melvin and Bren Simon
Comprehensive Cancer Center
Indianapolis, Indiana
888.600.4822 • www.cancer.iu.edu

Mayo Clinic Comprehensive Cancer Center
Phoenix/Scottsdale, Arizona
Jacksonville, Florida
Rochester, Minnesota
480.301.8000 • Arizona
904.953.0853 • Florida
507.538.3270 • Minnesota
mayoclinic.org/cancercenter

Memorial Sloan Kettering Cancer Center
New York, New York
800.525.2225 • mskcc.org

Moffitt Cancer Center
Tampa, Florida
888.663.3488 • moffitt.org

O'Neal Comprehensive Cancer Center at UAB
Birmingham, Alabama
800.822.0933 • uab.edu/onealcancercenter

Robert H. Lurie Comprehensive Cancer Center
of Northwestern University
Chicago, Illinois
866.587.4322 • cancer.northwestern.edu

Roswell Park Comprehensive Cancer Center
Buffalo, New York
877.275.7724 • roswellpark.org

Siteman Cancer Center at Barnes-Jewish Hospital
and Washington University School of Medicine
St. Louis, Missouri
800.600.3606 • siteman.wustl.edu

St. Jude Children's Research Hospital/
The University of Tennessee Health Science Center
Memphis, Tennessee
866.278.5833 • stjude.org
901.448.5500 • uthsc.edu

Stanford Cancer Institute
Stanford, California
877.668.7535 • cancer.stanford.edu

The Ohio State University Comprehensive Cancer Center -
James Cancer Hospital and Solove Research Institute
Columbus, Ohio
800.293.5066 • cancer.osu.edu

The Sidney Kimmel Comprehensive
Cancer Center at Johns Hopkins
Baltimore, Maryland
410.955.8964
www.hopkinskimmelcancercenter.org

The UChicago Medicine Comprehensive Cancer Center
Chicago, Illinois
773.702.1000 • uchicagomedicine.org/cancer

The University of Texas MD Anderson Cancer Center
Houston, Texas
844.269.5922 • mdanderson.org

UC Davis Comprehensive Cancer Center
Sacramento, California
916.734.5959 • 800.770.9261
health.ucdavis.edu/cancer

UC San Diego Moores Cancer Center
La Jolla, California
858.822.6100 • cancer.ucsd.edu

UCLA Jonsson Comprehensive Cancer Center
Los Angeles, California
310.825.5268 • uclahealth.org/cancer

UCSF Helen Diller Family
Comprehensive Cancer Center
San Francisco, California
800.689.8273 • cancer.ucsf.edu

University of Colorado Cancer Center
Aurora, Colorado
720.848.0300 • coloradocancercenter.org

University of Michigan Rogel Cancer Center
Ann Arbor, Michigan
800.865.1125 • rogelcancercenter.org

University of Wisconsin Carbone Cancer Center
Madison, Wisconsin
608.265.1700 • uwhealth.org/cancer

UT Southwestern Simmons
Comprehensive Cancer Center
Dallas, Texas
214.648.3111 • utsouthwestern.edu/simmons

Vanderbilt-Ingram Cancer Center
Nashville, Tennessee
877.936.8422 • vicc.org

Yale Cancer Center/Smilow Cancer Hospital
New Haven, Connecticut
855.4.SMILOW • yalecancercenter.org

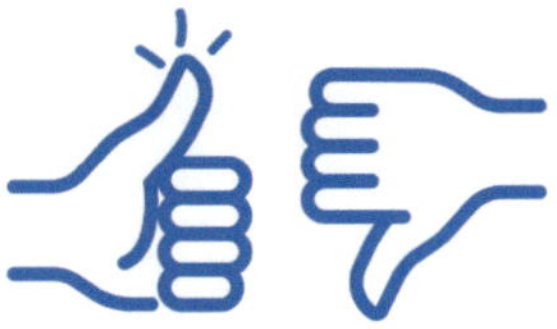

Let us know what you think!

Please take a moment to complete an online survey about the NCCN Guidelines for Patients.

NCCN.org/patients/response

Index

Made in the USA
Monee, IL
05 November 2026

67382283R00057